RISK MANAGEMENT FOR THE MEDICAL DEVICE INDUSTRY

A Guide Based On ISO 14971

Dr. Akash Sharma, Ms. Vriti Gamta and Mr. Gaurav Luthra

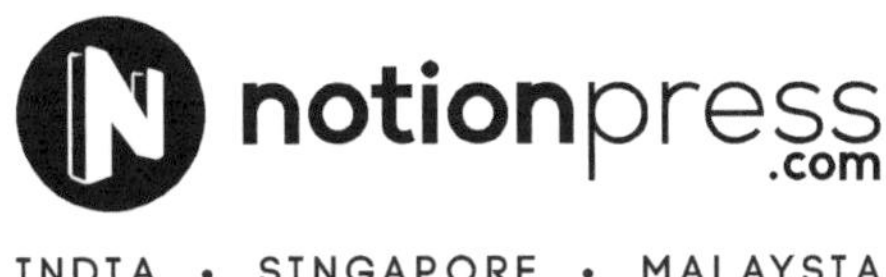

INDIA • SINGAPORE • MALAYSIA

ISBN 979-8-xxxxx-xxx-x

CONTENTS

PREFACE

Welcome to the **RISK MANAGEMENT FOR THE MEDICAL DEVICE INDUSTRY.** This book serves as a valuable resource for professionals involved in the development, manufacturing, and distribution of medical devices, as well as regulatory authorities and other stakeholders in the industry. The aim of this guide is to provide a thorough understanding of risk management principles and practices, with a specific focus on ISO 14971, the internationally recognized standard for risk management in medical devices. In today's dynamic healthcare landscape, ensuring the safety and efficacy of medical devices is of utmost importance. The complexity and diversity of medical devices, coupled with evolving regulatory requirements, necessitate a robust and systematic approach to risk management. Iso 14971 provides a structured framework that enables organizations to identify, analyze, evaluate, control, and monitor risks associated with medical devices throughout their life cycle. This guide is designed to demystify the principles and processes of risk management in the medical device industry. It takes a comprehensive approach, covering all the essential aspects of ISO 14971 and its application in the context of regulatory compliance, quality management systems, and global markets. Each section provides a detailed overview of the key concepts, supported by practical examples, tables, and diagrams to enhance understanding. Furthermore, this guide goes beyond ISO 14971 and explores the integration of risk management into the product life cycle, including product development, manufacturing, distribution, and post-market surveillance. It also addresses emerging trends and technologies such as unique device identification (UDI), artificial intelligence, internet of things (IoT), and cybersecurity, which have significant implications for risk management practices. Case studies and best practices presented throughout the guide offer real-world examples and insights, highlighting the application of risk management principles in different scenarios. The inclusion of templates, checklists, and glossary of terms in the appendices further enhances the practical value of this guide. It is important to note that while this guide provides a comprehensive overview of risk management in the medical device industry, it should be used in conjunction with the relevant regulatory requirements and guidelines specific to your region or country. Compliance with local regulations is essential for ensuring the safety and efficacy of medical devices. We hope that this guide will serve as a valuable reference and assist you in navigating the complex landscape of risk management in the medical device industry. By adopting a proactive and systematic approach to risk management, we can collectively contribute to the development of safe and effective medical devices that improve patient outcomes and advance healthcare globally.

ABOUT THE AUTHOR

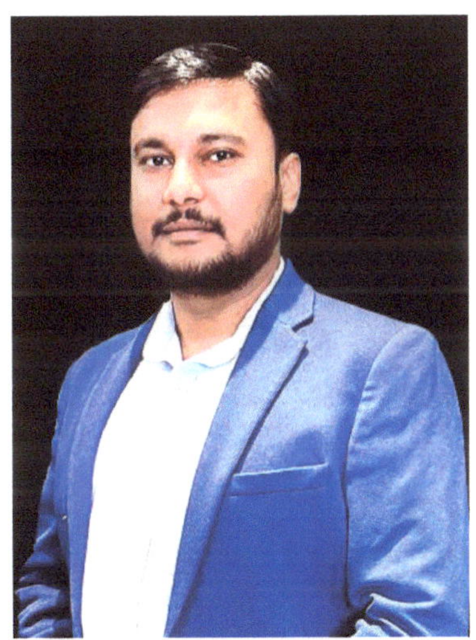

Dr. **Akash Sharma** is a highly accomplished professional in the field of Regulatory Affairs and Quality Management System for the medical device industry. With a strong academic background and extensive industry experience, Dr. Sharma brings a wealth of knowledge and expertise to the subject of Risk Management in this comprehensive guide. Dr. Sharma holds a Ph.D. & M.Tech in Mechanical Engineering. His research focus has been on the Application of Risk Management Principles in the Medical Device Industry, and he has published over 30 research papers in reputable journals.

Additionally, he has actively participated in more than 15 international conferences, where he has shared his insights and contributed to the advancements in the field. With a career spanning over seven years,

Dr. Sharma has gained valuable experience in regulatory affairs and quality management systems. He has a deep understanding of regulatory requirements, particularly in relation to the European Medical Device Regulation (EUMDR), CE certification and ISO 13485 for quality management systems. His expertise also extends to risk management, specifically in accordance with ISO 14971, the internationally recognized standard for managing risks associated with medical devices.

Currently serving as the Regulatory Affairs Manager and Management Representative at KAULMED PRIVATE LIMITED, Dr. Sharma plays a vital role in ensuring compliance with regulatory standards and driving quality initiatives within the organization. His hands-on experience in navigating the complexities of regulatory requirements and implementing effective risk management practices makes him a trusted authority in the field.

Dr. Sharma's passion for the medical device industry and his commitment to patient safety and product quality are evident in his work. Through this book, he shares his knowledge, practical insights, and best practices to guide professionals in the medical device industry towards successful risk management practices.

Dr. Akash Sharma's expertise, research contributions, and extensive industry experience make him a valuable resource for professionals seeking to enhance their understanding of risk management in the medical device industry. His dedication to excellence and continuous learning make him a trusted authority in the field.

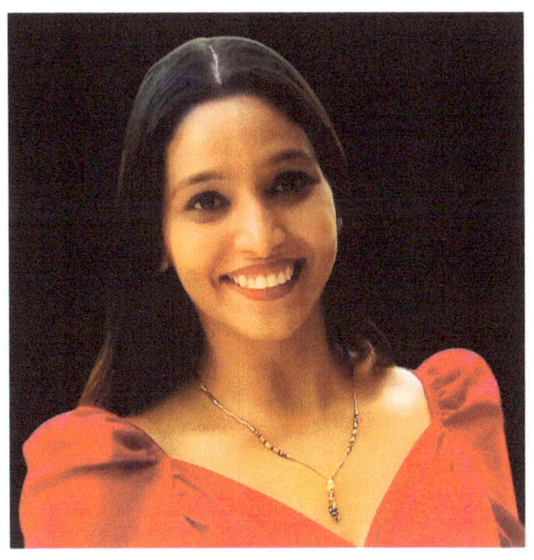

Vriti Gamta is a budding book author with a strong background in the healthcare industry. She holds a Master's degree in Pharmacy with a specialization in Drug Regulatory Affairs (DRA). With over four years of experience in Regulatory Affairs and Quality Management System, Vriti has established herself as an expert in navigating the complex regulatory landscape of the healthcare sector. Vriti's expertise lies in ensuring compliance with regulations and standards related to medical devices and pharmaceutical products. She is particularly knowledgeable in the European Union Medical Device Regulation (EUMDR), which sets out the requirements for placing medical devices on the market within the EU. In addition to her regulatory affairs proficiency, Vriti is well-versed in Quality Management Systems, specifically ISO 13485. This standard outlines the requirements for a comprehensive quality management system for the design, development, production, and distribution of medical devices.

Vriti has also developed a keen understanding of risk management principles, particularly ISO 14971. This international standard provides guidelines for identifying, evaluating, and controlling risks associated with medical devices throughout their lifecycle. Her commitment to advancing knowledge in her field is evident through her publication of three papers in international journals. These publications showcase her ability to conduct research, analyze data, and contribute to the scientific community within the healthcare industry.

Currently, Vriti holds the position of Regulatory Affairs Executive at KAULMED PRIVATE LIMITED, where she plays a crucial role in ensuring regulatory compliance and maintaining high-quality standards for the organization's medical devices and pharmaceutical products.

Vriti Gamta's combination of academic qualifications, extensive experience, and research contributions makes her a respected authority in Regulatory Affairs and Quality Management Systems within the healthcare industry. As a book author, she may reach a larger audience and impart her wisdom and insights, offering invaluable advice to both experts and enthusiasts.

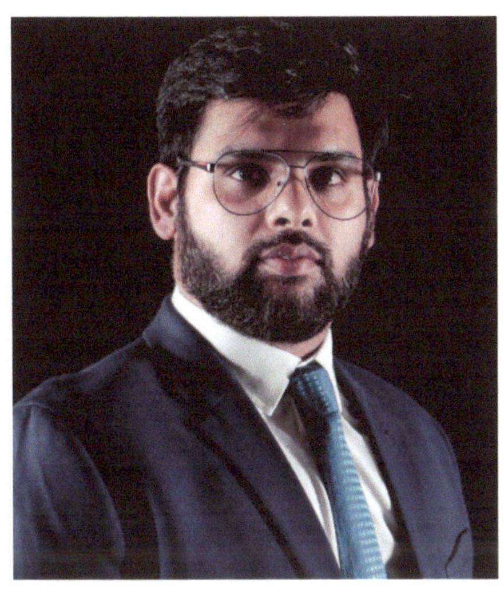

Gaurav **Luthra** is an accomplished author with a diverse range of experience in the medical device industry. With a career spanning 17 years, he has served as a Managing Director, leading and overseeing operations in the field. His extensive knowledge of manufacturing and new product development, regulatory affairs, quality management systems (QMS), and research and development has positioned him as an expert in his field. Throughout his career, Gaurav Luthra has contributed significantly through his research and publications. He has authored remarkable papers that have been published in renowned international journals.

As a Managing Director at KAULMED PRIVATE LIMITED, Gaurav Luthra has been responsible for driving innovation and spearheading research and development efforts within his organization. His focus on new product development has allowed him to stay at the forefront of technological advancements in the medical device industry, ensuring that his company remains competitive and continues to provide cutting-edge solutions. In addition to his expertise in manufacturing and product development. With a holistic approach to his work, Gaurav Luthra emphasizes the importance of quality management systems. He recognizes the significance of maintaining robust processes and procedures to ensure the consistent delivery of safe and effective medical devices. Through his experience, he has implemented and optimized QMS practices to meet the highest industry standards.

Gaurav Luthra's extensive experience and comprehensive understanding of the medical device industry make him an authoritative voice in his field. His dedication to research and development, combined with his expertise in manufacturing, regulatory affairs, and QMS, positions him as a valuable resource for professionals and researchers seeking insights into the medical device industry.

As an author, Gaurav Luthra can communicate complex concepts in a clear and concise manner. Overall, Gaurav Luthra's expertise, experience, and research contributions have solidified his reputation as a prominent figure in the medical device industry. Through his publications and managerial role, he continues to make significant contributions to the advancement and improvement of medical devices, ultimately benefiting patients and healthcare providers alike.

CHAPTER 1

INTRODUCTION TO RISK MANAGEMENT IN THE MEDICAL DEVICE INDUSTRY

Risk management plays a vital role in the medical device industry to ensure the safety and effectiveness of medical devices. It involves identifying, assessing, and mitigating potential risks associated with the development, manufacturing, distribution, and use of medical devices. The objective is to minimize the probability of harm to patients, users, and others while maximizing the benefits provided by the devices.

The complexity of medical devices, coupled with their potential impact on patient health, requires a systematic approach to risk management. It involves considering various factors, such as device design, manufacturing processes, intended use, and potential hazards that may arise during the device's lifecycle.

Regulatory bodies, such as the U.S. Food and Drug Administration (FDA) and the European Union Medical Device Regulation (MDR), impose specific requirements for risk management in the medical device industry. Compliance with international standards, such as ISO 14971, is often expected to demonstrate adherence to recognized best practices in risk management.

By adopting a systematic and proactive approach to risk management, medical device manufacturers can enhance the safety, quality, and performance of their devices while ensuring regulatory compliance and customer satisfaction.

1.1 OVERVIEW OF RISK MANAGEMENT

Risk management is a systematic and ongoing process of identifying, assessing, prioritizing, and mitigating risks to achieve objectives and minimize potential negative impacts. It is a fundamental practice utilized by organizations across various industries to proactively address uncertainties and make informed decisions. Figure 1.1 shows the overview of Risk Management Process.

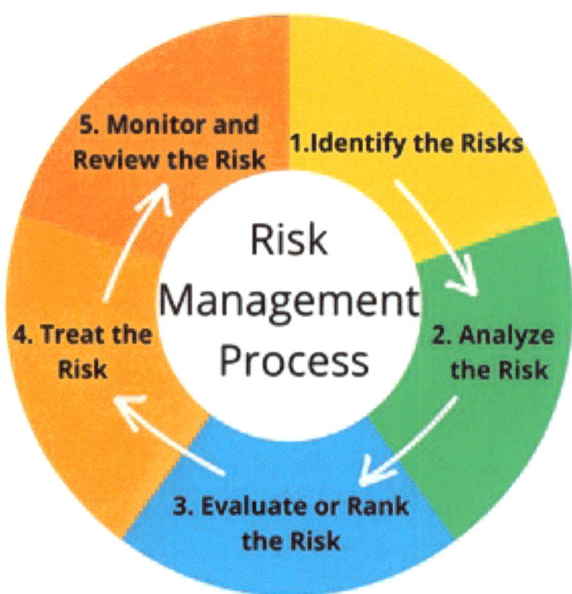

FIGURE 1.1- OVERVIEW OF RISK MANAGEMENT PROCESS

The **key elements** of risk management include:

1. **Risk Identification:** The process of recognizing and understanding potential risks that may affect the achievement of objectives. This involves systematically identifying potential risks by considering internal and external factors that could impact the organization's objectives. It can be done through techniques such as brainstorming, checklists, historical data analysis, expert opinions, and scenario analysis. Effective risk identification ensures that a wide range of risks is considered, enabling the organization to develop appropriate risk response strategies.

2. **Risk Assessment:** Risk assessment involves analyzing identified risks to understand their likelihood and potential impact. This step helps prioritize risks based on their significance, allowing organizations to focus their resources on managing the most critical risks. Risk assessment often involves using qualitative and quantitative methods to evaluate risks, such as probability and impact matrices, risk scoring, and statistical analysis.

3. **Risk Analysis:** Risk analysis delves deeper into the nature and characteristics of identified risks. It aims to understand the causes, drivers, and potential interdependencies among risks. Conducting a detailed examination of identified risks to gain a deeper understanding of their causes, triggers, and potential interdependencies. This analysis helps in developing effective risk response strategies. Various techniques can be used, including root cause analysis, fault tree analysis, failure mode and effect analysis (FMEA), and SWOT analysis. By conducting thorough risk analysis, organizations gain a better understanding of the underlying factors contributing to risks and can develop more effective risk mitigation strategies.

4. **Risk Evaluation:** Risk evaluation involves assessing the significance of risks in relation to the organization's objectives and risk appetite. It requires comparing the assessed risks against predefined criteria or thresholds to determine their acceptability. This step helps decision-makers understand the potential impact of risks on the organization's ability to achieve its goals and make informed choices regarding risk treatment options.

5. **Risk Treatment:** Risk treatment is the process of developing and implementing strategies to address identified risks. The goal is to reduce the likelihood or impact of risks to an acceptable level. Risk treatment options may include implementing controls, improving processes, transferring risks to third parties through insurance or contracts, or accepting certain risks while actively monitoring them. The chosen risk treatment strategies should align with the organization's risk management objectives and risk tolerance levels.

6. **Risk Monitoring and Review:** Continuous monitoring and review of risks are essential to ensure that risk management remains effective and relevant over time. It involves regularly assessing the performance of risk controls, tracking changes in risk profiles, and identifying emerging risks. Risk monitoring enables organizations to take proactive measures, adjust risk treatments if necessary, and maintain an up-to-date understanding of their risk landscape.

7. **Risk Communication:** Effective risk communication is crucial for promoting a risk-aware culture and ensuring stakeholders have the necessary information to make informed decisions. This involves clear and timely communication of risks, risk management strategies, and risk-related performance to relevant stakeholders. Transparent communication builds trust, encourages collaboration, and facilitates the integration of risk management into organizational decision-making processes.

8. **Documentation and Record-Keeping:** Documentation serves as a record of the organization's risk management activities. It helps demonstrate compliance with regulations, provides evidence of due diligence, and supports accountability. Comprehensive documentation includes risk assessments, risk treatment plans, risk monitoring reports, and the rationale behind decisions made. Proper record-keeping ensures that the organization maintains a historical reference for future analysis, audits, and improvement initiatives.

Risk management is not a one-time activity but an ongoing and iterative process that should be embedded within an organization's culture and operations. It helps organizations identify potential threats and opportunities, make informed decisions, and improve resilience and performance in the face of uncertainties. By embracing a robust risk management approach, organizations can anticipate and respond to potential risks more effectively, seize opportunities, and optimize their performance while minimizing potential disruptions. Risk management should be an integral part of organizational processes and systems to foster a culture that values risk awareness, promotes informed decision-making, and drives sustainable success.

1.2 IMPORTANCE OF RISK MANAGEMENT IN THE MEDICAL DEVICE INDUSTRY

Risk management holds significant importance in the medical device industry due to the critical nature of medical devices and the potential impact they have on patient safety and well-being. Here are some key reasons why risk management is crucial in this industry (Figure 1.2):

1. **Patient Safety:** The primary objective of risk management in the medical device industry is to ensure patient safety. By systematically identifying and assessing potential risks, manufacturers can take appropriate measures to mitigate or eliminate those risks, reducing the likelihood of harm to patients. This proactive approach helps protect patients from potential hazards associated with medical devices.

2. **Regulatory Compliance:** The medical device industry is subject to strict regulatory requirements to ensure product safety and efficacy. Regulatory authorities, such as the FDA in the United States or the European Medicines Agency (EMA) in Europe, expect manufacturers to have robust risk management processes in place. Compliance with regulatory standards and guidelines, such as ISO 14971, demonstrates an organization's commitment to quality and safety, facilitating market access and regulatory approvals.

3. **Product Liability and Legal Considerations:** Medical device manufacturers face potential legal and financial risks if their products cause harm or are involved in adverse events. Implementing effective risk management practices helps minimize these risks by identifying and addressing potential product-related hazards and vulnerabilities. Adequate risk management demonstrates due diligence, potentially reducing legal liability and associated costs.

4. **Reputation and Brand Protection:** A product recall or safety issue can severely damage a medical device manufacturer's reputation and

brand image. Proactive risk management helps prevent or minimize such incidents, safeguarding the company's reputation and maintaining customer trust. Organizations that prioritize risk management and prioritize patient safety are more likely to establish a positive brand reputation in the industry.

5. **Improved Product Quality and Reliability:** Risk management practices can contribute to the development of high-quality and reliable medical devices. By identifying potential risks and implementing appropriate risk control measures, manufacturers can enhance product design, manufacturing processes, and overall quality. This, in turn, improves product performance, reduces failure rates, and enhances customer satisfaction.

6. **Cost Reduction and Efficiency:** Effective risk management can lead to cost savings by avoiding potential liabilities, recalls, or product failures. By identifying risks early in the product development phase, manufacturers can proactively address them, reducing the need for costly rework, modifications, or redesigns. Additionally, efficient risk management processes streamline decision-making, improve resource allocation, and optimize overall operational efficiency.

7. **Post-Market Surveillance and Continuous Improvement:** Risk management is not limited to the pre-market phase but extends throughout the entire lifecycle of medical devices. It involves post-market surveillance activities, including monitoring adverse events, analyzing feedback from users, and implementing necessary corrective and preventive actions. This feedback loop enables continuous improvement, allowing organizations to respond to emerging risks, enhance product safety, and meet evolving regulatory requirements.

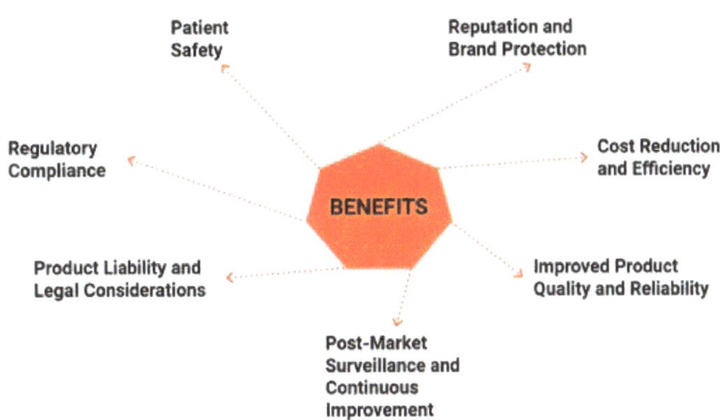

FIGURE 1.2- WHY RISK MANAGEMENT?

Overall, risk management is a critical component of ensuring patient safety, regulatory compliance, and the long-term success of medical device manufacturers. By proactively identifying and managing risks, organizations can develop high-quality, reliable, and safe medical devices that improve patient outcomes and maintain stakeholder confidence.

1.3 ISO 14971: OVERVIEW AND PURPOSE

ISO 14971 is an international standard that provides guidance on risk management for medical devices. It sets out principles and processes to identify, analyze, evaluate, and manage risks associated with medical devices throughout their lifecycle. The standard aims to ensure the safety and effectiveness of medical devices by addressing potential hazards and minimizing the risks they pose to patients, users, and others.

Here's an overview of ISO 14971 and its purpose:

1. **Scope:** ISO 14971 applies to the entire lifecycle of a medical device, from its conception and design to manufacturing, distribution, use, and disposal. It applies to all types of medical devices, including active devices, non-active devices, and in vitro diagnostic devices.

2. **Risk Management Framework:** ISO 14971 provides a comprehensive risk management framework that outlines the key steps and activities involved in managing risks associated with medical devices. It emphasizes a systematic and iterative approach to risk management that should be integrated into the organization's quality management system.

3. **Risk Management Process:** The standard outlines a step-by-step process for risk management, including risk identification, risk analysis, risk evaluation, risk control, and overall risk management review. This process enables manufacturers to identify and evaluate potential hazards, estimate the associated risks, implement appropriate risk control measures, and continuously monitor and improve the risk management process.

4. **Risk Management File:** ISO 14971 emphasizes the importance of maintaining a risk management file that documents all risk management activities and decisions related to the medical device. The file serves as a comprehensive record of risk assessments, risk control measures, risk management plans, and risk management reports, providing evidence of compliance with the standard.

5. **Risk Benefit Analysis:** ISO 14971 emphasizes the need to balance the risks associated with a medical device against its intended benefits. It requires manufacturers to conduct a risk-benefit analysis to evaluate the overall benefit-risk profile of the device. This analysis helps ensure that the risks associated with the device are justified by the benefits it provides.

6. **Post-Market Surveillance:** The standard recognizes the importance of post-market surveillance in monitoring the performance and safety of medical devices. It emphasizes the need for manufacturers to have processes in place to collect and analyze post-market data, including adverse events and feedback from users, to identify and address emerging risks.

The **purpose** of ISO 14971 is to provide a harmonized and systematic approach to risk management for medical devices. It helps manufacturers establish a proactive risk management system that ensures patient safety, regulatory compliance, and the effective management of risks throughout the entire lifecycle of a medical device. By following the principles and processes outlined in ISO 14971, organizations can enhance their risk management capabilities and make informed decisions to minimize potential harm and optimize the benefit-risk balance of their medical devices.

The purpose of ISO 14971 is multifaceted and encompasses several key objectives.

1. **Ensuring Patient Safety:** The primary purpose of ISO 14971 is to ensure patient safety by minimizing the risks associated with medical devices. It provides a systematic approach to identifying potential hazards, assessing risks, and implementing appropriate risk control measures. By following the standard's guidelines, manufacturers can mitigate or eliminate risks that could harm patients, users, or others.

2. **Regulatory Compliance:** ISO 14971 serves as a recognized framework for risk management in the medical device industry. Compliance with the standard is often a regulatory requirement imposed by authorities such as the FDA in the United States, the European Medicines Agency (EMA) in Europe, and other regulatory bodies globally. Adhering to ISO 14971 helps manufacturers demonstrate compliance with regulatory expectations, facilitating market access and regulatory approvals.

3. **Integration with Quality Management Systems:** ISO 14971 emphasizes the integration of risk management into an organization's quality management system (QMS). The purpose is to establish a cohesive and comprehensive approach to managing risks that aligns with the organization's overall quality objectives and processes. By integrating risk management with the QMS, manufacturers can ensure a systematic and consistent approach to risk management across all stages of the medical device lifecycle.

4. **Facilitating Decision-Making:** ISO 14971 provides a structured and transparent process for risk management, which supports informed decision-making. It helps manufacturers evaluate the significance of risks and the effectiveness of risk control measures, facilitating decisions on risk acceptance, risk mitigation strategies, and product development or modification. The standard's risk management process assists organizations in making evidence-based decisions regarding their medical devices.

5. **Enhancing Product Development:** ISO 14971 encourages a proactive approach to risk management from the early stages of product development. By considering potential risks during the design and development phase, manufacturers can incorporate safety features and design controls that reduce risks and enhance the overall safety and performance of the medical device. This proactive risk management approach contributes to the development of high-quality and reliable medical devices.

6. **Supporting Continuous Improvement:** ISO 14971 emphasizes the importance of monitoring and reviewing risk management processes and outcomes. By regularly assessing the effectiveness of risk controls and collecting post-market data, manufacturers can identify new risks, emerging hazards, and areas for improvement. This supports a culture of continuous improvement, enabling organizations to refine their risk management strategies and enhance the safety and effectiveness of their medical devices over time.

1.4 STRUCTURE OF ISO 14971

ISO 14971 is structured into several sections that outline the principles, processes, and requirements for risk management of medical devices. The standard comprises the following main sections:

1. **Scope:** This section provides a brief description of the standard's scope, stating that ISO 14971 applies to the entire lifecycle of a medical device, from its conception to disposal.

2. **Normative References:** This section lists other relevant standards and documents that are referenced in ISO 14971 and should be considered when implementing risk management processes for medical devices.

3. **Terms and Definitions:** This section provides definitions of key terms used throughout the standard to ensure a common understanding of the terminology related to risk management in the context of medical devices.

4. **Risk Management Process:** This section forms the core of ISO 14971 and outlines the step-by-step risk management process to be followed. It includes the following main steps:

   a. **Risk Management Planning:** This step involves establishing the scope, objectives, and activities of the risk management process, as well as defining the roles and responsibilities of individuals involved.

   b. **Risk Identification:** This step focuses on systematically identifying and documenting potential hazards associated with the medical device and its intended use. It includes considering all possible hazards, including those arising from device malfunctions, use errors, and external factors.

   c. **Risk Analysis:** In this step, the identified risks are evaluated by considering their likelihood of occurrence and potential consequences. Various methods, such as qualitative or quantitative analysis, can be used to assess the risks.

   d. **Risk Evaluation:** This step involves comparing the estimated risks against predefined criteria, such as acceptable risk levels or the organization's risk tolerance. The purpose is to determine the significance of risks and prioritize them for further action.

   e. **Risk Control:** In this step, risk control measures are developed and implemented to reduce risks to an acceptable level. The standard emphasizes the concept of a risk control hierarchy, where risk reduction measures are implemented in a systematic order, starting with inherent safety measures and progressing to protective measures and information for safety.

f. **Residual Risk Evaluation:** After implementing risk controls, the remaining risks are re-evaluated to assess their acceptability and ensure that they have been reduced to an acceptable level.

g. **Risk Management Review:** This step involves periodically reviewing and reassessing the effectiveness of the risk management process, including the suitability and adequacy of implemented risk controls. It also includes assessing the need for further action, such as updating risk management documentation or initiating corrective measures.

5. **Annexes:** ISO 14971 includes informative annexes that provide additional guidance and information related to specific topics. The annexes cover areas such as risk management principles, risk management system, risk management file, and examples of risk management techniques (as shown in Table 1.1).

It is important to note that ISO 14971 provides a framework and guidance for risk management, but it does not prescribe specific methods or tools to be used. The standard allows organizations flexibility in implementing risk management processes that are appropriate for their specific context and medical devices.

TABLE 1.1: ANNEXES

Annex Number	Title
Annex A	Risk Management Principles
Annex B	Risk Management System
Annex C	Risk Management File
Annex D	Example of a Risk Management Process
Annex E	Example of a Risk Management Plan
Annex F	Example of a Risk Management Report
Annex G	Example of Risk Management Documentation
Annex H	Example of a Risk Management Record
Annex I	Example of a Risk Analysis Technique: Preliminary Hazard Analysis

Annex Number	Title
Annex J	Example of a Risk Analysis Technique: Failure Mode and Effects Analysis
Annex K	Example of a Risk Analysis Technique: Fault Tree Analysis

1.5 APPLICABILITY OF ISO 14971 TO THE MEDICAL DEVICE INDUSTRY

ISO 14971 is specifically designed for and applicable to the medical device industry. It provides guidance and requirements for the implementation of risk management processes throughout the lifecycle of medical devices. Here's a closer look at the applicability of ISO 14971 to the medical device industry (as summarized in Figure 1.3):

1. **Medical Device Types:** ISO 14971 applies to all types of medical devices, including both active and non-active devices, as well as in vitro diagnostic devices. It covers a wide range of medical devices, such as diagnostic equipment, implantable devices, surgical instruments, monitoring devices, and more.

2. **Lifecycle Stages:** The standard applies to the entire lifecycle of a medical device, from its conception and development to manufacturing, distribution, use, and eventual disposal. It emphasizes the importance of integrating risk management activities at each stage to ensure the safety and effectiveness of the device.

3. **Risk Management Framework:** ISO 14971 provides a comprehensive framework for risk management specific to the medical device industry. It outlines the principles, processes, and requirements for identifying, analyzing, evaluating, and managing risks associated with medical devices. The standard helps manufacturers establish a systematic and consistent approach to risk management, ensuring that potential hazards and risks are addressed throughout the device's lifecycle.

4. **Regulatory Compliance:** Compliance with ISO 14971 is often a regulatory requirement imposed by authorities such as the FDA in

the United States, the European Medicines Agency (EMA) in Europe, and other regulatory bodies worldwide. Regulatory bodies expect medical device manufacturers to demonstrate adherence to recognized international standards, such as ISO 14971, as part of their regulatory submissions and conformity assessment processes.

5. **Integration with Quality Management Systems:** ISO 14971 emphasizes the integration of risk management with an organization's quality management system (QMS). It aligns risk management activities with existing quality processes, ensuring a comprehensive and cohesive approach to managing risks. This integration enables manufacturers to effectively manage risks while maintaining compliance with other quality standards, such as ISO 13485.

6. **Post-Market Surveillance:** ISO 14971 recognizes the importance of post-market surveillance in monitoring the performance and safety of medical devices. It emphasizes the need for manufacturers to establish processes for collecting and analyzing post-market data, including adverse events, complaints, and feedback from users. This data plays a crucial role in identifying and addressing emerging risks and ensuring continuous improvement of the device's safety profile.

7. **Harmonization and Consistency:** ISO 14971 provides a globally recognized framework for risk management in the medical device industry. Its guidelines and requirements help establish a common language and understanding of risk management practices across different geographical regions. This harmonization facilitates consistency in risk management approaches, promoting the safe and effective use of medical devices worldwide.

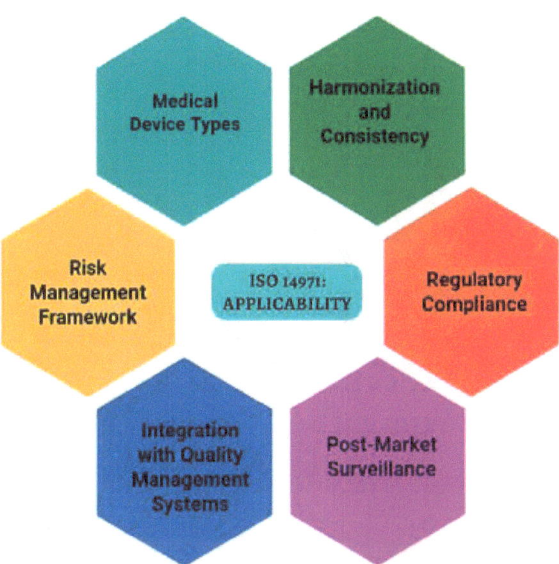

FIGURE 1.3- ISO 14971: APPLICABILITY

To summarize, ISO 14971 is highly applicable to the medical device industry. Its guidance and requirements help manufacturers establish robust risk management processes to ensure the safety and effectiveness of medical devices throughout their lifecycle. Compliance with ISO 14971 demonstrates a commitment to patient safety, regulatory requirements, and the overall quality of medical devices.

CHAPTER 2

REGULATORY FRAMEWORK AND STANDARDS

The medical device industry operates within a regulatory framework that sets forth requirements and standards to ensure the safety, efficacy, and quality of medical devices. The regulatory framework varies across countries and regions, but there are some key components and standards that are commonly followed. Here's an overview of the regulatory framework and standards in the medical device industry:

1. **Regulatory authorities:** each country or region has its own regulatory authority responsible for overseeing the medical device industry. for example, the food and drug administration (FDA) in the united states, the European medicines agency (EMA) in europe, and the pharmaceuticals and medical devices agency (PMDA) in japan. these regulatory authorities establish and enforce regulations to protect public health and ensure the safety and effectiveness of medical devices.

2. **Regulations and directives:** regulatory bodies issue regulations and directives that outline legal requirements for medical devices. these regulations cover various aspects, such as product classification, pre-market approval processes, post-market surveillance, labeling and packaging requirements, and manufacturing practices. examples of regulations include the medical device regulation (MDR) in the European union and the medical devices act (MDA) in the united states.

3. **International standards:** international standards provide guidance and best practices for various aspects of medical device development,

manufacturing, and quality management. standards are often used by regulatory authorities as a reference for assessing compliance. some of the prominent international standards in the medical device industry include:

- **ISO 13485:** This standard specifies requirements for a quality management system specific to the medical device industry. It sets forth criteria for designing, manufacturing, and distributing medical devices while ensuring compliance with regulatory requirements.

- **ISO 14971:** As discussed earlier, ISO 14971 focuses on risk management for medical devices. It provides a framework and guidance for identifying, evaluating, and controlling risks associated with medical devices throughout their lifecycle.

- **IEC 60601:** This series of standards addresses the safety and performance of medical electrical equipment. It covers a wide range of devices, including diagnostic equipment, patient monitoring systems, and therapeutic devices.

4. **Harmonization And Mutual Recognition:** To facilitate global trade and streamline regulatory processes, there are initiatives to harmonize regulations and promote mutual recognition of regulatory decisions. For example, the Global Harmonization Task Force (GHTF) was established to harmonize regulatory requirements across different regions. The GHTF has now transitioned to the International Medical Device Regulators Forum (IMDRF), which continues to work toward regulatory convergence and cooperation.

5. **Post-market Surveillance:** Regulatory authorities emphasize post-market surveillance to monitor the safety and performance of medical devices once they are on the market. Manufacturers are required to establish processes for collecting and analyzing post-market data, such as adverse event reports, complaints, and recalls. This information is vital for identifying and addressing any safety issues or emerging risks associated with medical devices.

It's important for medical device manufacturers to stay updated with the regulatory framework and standards applicable to their target markets. Adhering to the regulatory requirements and implementing relevant standards is essential for obtaining regulatory approvals, ensuring compliance, and demonstrating the safety and quality of medical devices.

2.1 GLOBAL REGULATORY REQUIREMENTS FOR MEDICAL DEVICES

Global regulatory requirements for medical devices can vary between countries and regions. However, there are some key regulatory bodies and frameworks that oversee the safety, efficacy, and quality of medical devices worldwide. Here's an overview of the global regulatory requirements for medical devices:

1. **United States:**
   - **Food and Drug Administration (FDA):** The FDA regulates medical devices in the United States under the Federal Food, Drug, and Cosmetic Act (FD&C Act). Medical devices are classified into different classes (Class I, II, and III) based on their level of risk, and manufacturers must adhere to pre-market approval processes, such as 510(k) clearance or Pre-market Approval (PMA).

2. **European Union:**
   - **European Medical Devices Regulation (MDR):** The MDR is a comprehensive regulatory framework that sets requirements for medical devices in the European Union (EU). It covers device classification, conformity assessment procedures, post-market surveillance, and labeling and packaging requirements. It also introduced a Unique Device Identification (UDI) system and stricter requirements for clinical evaluation and post-market clinical follow-up.

3. **Canada:**
   - **Health Canada:** Health Canada regulates medical devices in Canada under the Medical Devices Regulations. Manufacturers must obtain

a Medical Device License (MDL) before selling their products in the Canadian market. The regulatory requirements include device classification, quality management system certification, and post-market surveillance obligations.

4. **Japan:**
   - **Pharmaceuticals and Medical Devices Agency (PMDA):** The PMDA oversees medical device regulations in Japan. Manufacturers must comply with the Pharmaceutical Affairs Law (PAL) and undergo pre-market certification processes, such as Shonin (marketing authorization) or Ninsho (notification). Japan has unique requirements for clinical trials and post-market safety management.

5. **Australia:**
   - **Therapeutic Goods Administration (TGA):** The TGA regulates medical devices in Australia under the Therapeutic Goods Act. Medical devices are classified into different risk categories (Class I, IIa, IIb, III, and AIMD), and manufacturers must obtain Conformity Assessment Certification before marketing their devices in Australia. The TGA also introduced the Australian Register of Therapeutic Goods (ARTG) for device registration.

6. **China:**
   - **National Medical Products Administration (NMPA):** The NMPA regulates medical devices in China. Manufacturers must obtain product registration certificates before marketing their devices in China. The regulatory requirements include device classification, clinical trial approvals, and compliance with Good Manufacturing Practice (GMP) standards.

7. **International Harmonization:**
   - **International Medical Device Regulators Forum (IMDRF):** The IMDRF is an international forum that aims to harmonize medical device regulations across countries. The IMDRF develops

guidelines and frameworks to promote regulatory convergence and cooperation, with a focus on areas such as risk management, clinical evaluation, and post-market surveillance.

It's important to note that each country or region may have its own specific requirements, and regulatory frameworks can evolve over time. Medical device manufacturers should consult the relevant regulatory authorities and stay updated with the specific requirements applicable to their target markets.

2.2 RELATIONSHIP BETWEEN ISO 14971 AND REGULATORY COMPLIANCE

ISO 14971, the international standard for risk management of medical devices, plays a crucial role in regulatory compliance for the medical device industry. The relationship between ISO 14971 and regulatory compliance is described below with the help of Figure 2.1:

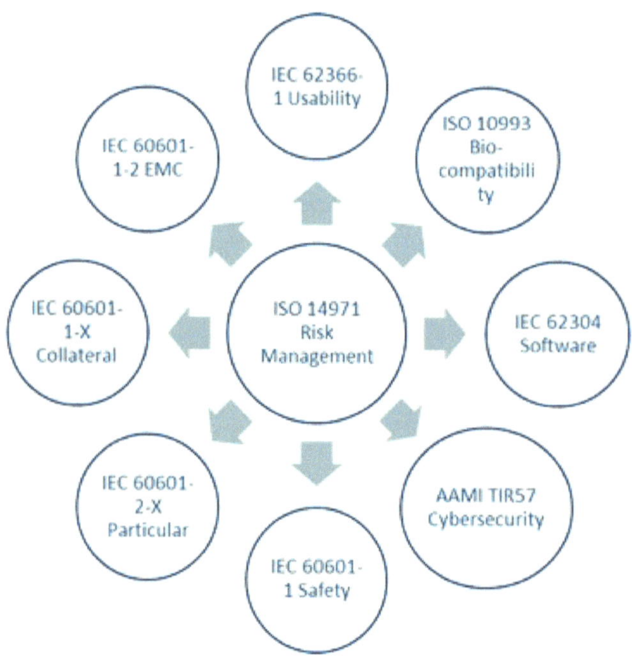

FIGURE 2.1: RELATIONSHIP BETWEEN ISO 14971 AND REGULATORY COMPLIANCE

1. **Alignment With Regulatory Requirements:** ISO 14971 is designed to align with regulatory requirements and expectations for risk management in the medical device industry. It provides a systematic and comprehensive framework that helps manufacturers address and fulfill regulatory obligations related to risk management. By implementing ISO 14971, medical device manufacturers can demonstrate their commitment to meeting regulatory requirements.

2. **Regulatory Recognition:** Regulatory authorities worldwide recognize ISO 14971 as a widely accepted and globally harmonized standard for risk management in the medical device industry. They often refer to ISO 14971 as a benchmark for assessing the adequacy of a manufacturer's risk management processes during regulatory inspections and audits. Compliance with ISO 14971 can facilitate regulatory approvals and enhance the credibility of a manufacturer's risk management practices.

3. **Common Language And Approach:** ISO 14971 provides a common language and approach for risk management across the medical device industry. By adhering to ISO 14971, manufacturers can communicate and collaborate effectively with regulatory authorities, notified bodies, and other stakeholders involved in the regulatory process. It promotes consistency and mutual understanding in risk management practices, making it easier to navigate regulatory requirements.

4. **Integration With Regulatory Processes:** ISO 14971 emphasizes the integration of risk management activities into the overall regulatory processes of medical device manufacturers. It encourages manufacturers to incorporate risk management throughout the product lifecycle, including pre-market activities such as design, development, and clinical evaluation, as well as post-market activities such as vigilance reporting and post-market surveillance. This integration ensures that risk management is an integral part of regulatory compliance efforts.

5. **Evidence Of Compliance:** ISO 14971 provides a structured approach for documenting risk management activities and maintaining a risk management file. This documentation serves as valuable evidence

of compliance with regulatory requirements. It helps manufacturers demonstrate that they have identified potential risks, assessed their significance, implemented appropriate risk controls, and evaluated the effectiveness of those controls. This evidence is vital during regulatory submissions, audits, and inspections.

6. **Continuous Improvement:** ISO 14971 promotes a lifecycle approach to risk management, emphasizing the need for continuous monitoring, evaluation, and improvement of risk management processes. This aligns with regulatory expectations for post-market surveillance, feedback analysis, and ongoing risk assessment. By implementing ISO 14971, manufacturers can establish mechanisms for collecting post-market data, evaluating emerging risks, and implementing necessary corrective actions to ensure the ongoing safety and effectiveness of their devices.

ISO 14971 and regulatory compliance are closely linked. ISO 14971 provides a comprehensive framework for risk management in the medical device industry, which aligns with regulatory requirements, facilitates regulatory recognition, and supports effective integration of risk management into regulatory processes. Compliance with ISO 14971 helps manufacturers meet regulatory obligations, enhance product safety, and demonstrate their commitment to patient safety and regulatory compliance.

2.3 KEY STANDARDS AND GUIDELINES RELATED TO RISK MANAGEMENT IN MEDICAL DEVICES

There are several key standards and guidelines related to risk management in medical devices. These standards provide guidance and best practices for implementing effective risk management processes in the medical device industry. Some of the notable standards and guidelines are:

1. **ISO 14971:** This is the international standard for medical device risk management. It provides a comprehensive framework for identifying, evaluating, and controlling risks associated with medical devices throughout their lifecycle. ISO 14971 outlines the principles, processes, and activities necessary for effective risk management, including risk assessment, risk control, and risk communication.

2. **IEC 62304:** This standard focuses on the software lifecycle processes for medical device software. It provides guidance on the development, maintenance, and risk management of software used in medical devices. IEC 62304 outlines the activities and documentation required for software development, verification, and validation, with an emphasis on risk management specific to software.

3. **ISO 13485:** Although ISO 13485 is a quality management system standard, it includes requirements related to risk management. ISO 13485 specifies the criteria for designing, developing, manufacturing, and maintaining medical devices. It emphasizes the need for a systematic approach to risk management throughout the organization and across the product lifecycle.

4. **IEC 60601 series:** This series of standards covers the safety and performance of medical electrical equipment. The standards within IEC 60601 provide specific requirements for different types of medical devices, addressing electrical safety, electromagnetic compatibility, and other risk-related considerations. The standards in this series are widely used for medical devices incorporating electrical or electronic components.

5. **FDA Guidance Documents:** The U.S. Food and Drug Administration (FDA) has issued various guidance documents related to risk management in medical devices. These documents provide additional interpretation and recommendations for complying with regulatory requirements. Examples include the FDA's "General Principles of Software Validation" and the "Guidance on Design Control for Medical Device Manufacturers."

6. **MEDDEV Guidelines:** The European Commission's Medical Device Vigilance System (MEDDEV) guidelines provide guidance on the interpretation and implementation of the European medical device regulations. MEDDEV 2.7/1 rev. 4 specifically focuses on clinical evaluation and includes guidance on risk management aspects related to clinical evaluation of medical devices.

7. **AAMI TIR57:** The Association for the Advancement of Medical Instrumentation (AAMI) Technical Information Report (TIR) 57 provides guidance on the application of ISO 14971 to medical device cybersecurity. It helps manufacturers understand and manage the risks associated with the cybersecurity of medical devices.

These are just a few examples of the key standards and guidelines related to risk management in the medical device industry. It's important for medical device manufacturers to consult and adhere to the applicable standards and guidelines based on their specific product types, markets, and regulatory requirements.

RISK MANAGEMENT PROCESS ACCORDING TO ISO 14971

The risk management process according to ISO 14971 follows a systematic approach to identify, evaluate, control, and monitor risks associated with medical devices. Here is a simplified outline of the risk management process (as discussed in Table 3.1 and Figure 3.1 and 3.2):

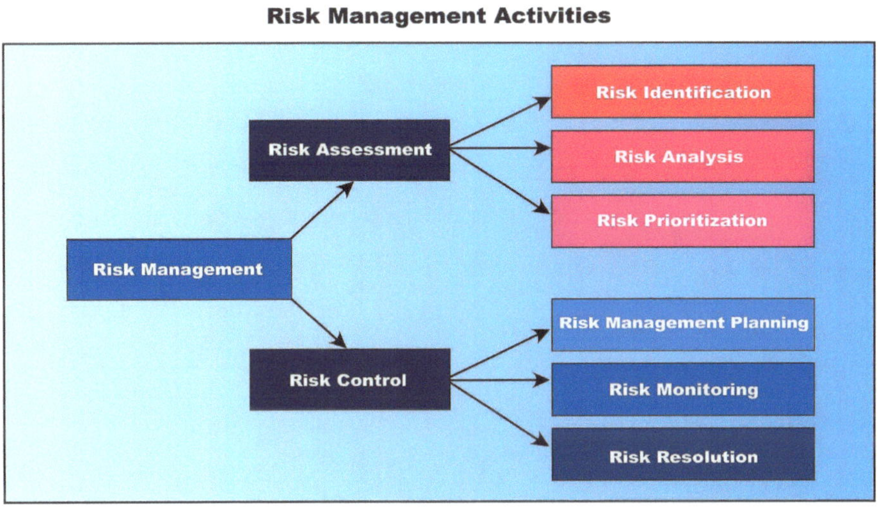

Risk Management Activities

FIGURE 3.1: RISK MANAGEMENT ACTIVITIES

TABLE 3.1: RISK MANAGEMENT PROCESS ACCORDING TO ISO 14971

S. NO.	STEPS	DESCRIPTION
1	Risk Management Planning	✦ Establish the scope and objectives of the risk management process. ✦ Define roles and responsibilities of individuals involved. ✦ Determine the methods and tools to be used for risk management.
2	Risk Analysis	✦ Identify potential hazards associated with the medical device. ✦ Evaluate the likelihood and severity of harm that could result from each hazard. ✦ Determine the risk priority by considering the probability of occurrence and the potential severity of harm.
3	Risk Evaluation	✦ Compare the identified risks against predetermined acceptability criteria. ✦ Assess the need for risk reduction measures based on the acceptability of the risks. ✦ Determine whether the residual risks are acceptable or further action is required.
4	Risk Control	✦ Implement risk control measures to reduce risks to an acceptable level. ✦ Consider the principles of the hierarchy of controls (elimination, substitution, engineering controls, administrative controls, and personal protective equipment). ✦ Document the risk control measures and their effectiveness in reducing or mitigating risks.

5	Residual Risk Evaluation (risk Acceptability)	✦ Evaluate the remaining risks after implementing risk control measures. ✦ Determine whether the residual risks are acceptable based on the acceptability criteria. ✦ If necessary, revise risk control measures to reduce the risks further.
6	Risk Management Review	✦ Review the overall risk management process to ensure its effectiveness. ✦ Consider feedback from post-market surveillance and other sources to identify any new risks or changes in existing risks. ✦ Update the risk management file and documentation as necessary.
7	Risk Management Report	✦ Prepare a risk management report that summarizes the risk management process, including the identified hazards, risk evaluation results, risk control measures, and residual risks. ✦ Include any assumptions, limitations, and uncertainties associated with the risk assessment.
8	Production And Post-market Activities	✦ Implement risk management activities throughout the device lifecycle, including manufacturing, post-market surveillance, and vigilance reporting. ✦ Continuously monitor and evaluate the device's performance and safety information to identify any potential new risks or changes in existing risks. ✦ Take appropriate actions to address identified risks, such as implementing corrective and preventive measures.

3.1 RISK MANAGEMENT PLANNING

Risk Management Planning is the initial step in the risk management process according to ISO 14971. It involves establishing a plan that outlines the approach, objectives, and activities for managing risks associated with a medical device. Here are the key elements of risk management planning:

1. **Define the Scope:** Clearly define the scope of the risk management process, specifying the medical device or product family to be considered. This helps ensure that the risk management activities are focused on the relevant aspects of the device.

2. **Establish Objectives:** Set clear objectives for the risk management process. These objectives should align with the organization's overall goals and regulatory requirements. Objectives may include ensuring patient safety, complying with applicable regulations, and minimizing risks to an acceptable level.

3. **Identify Stakeholders:** Identify the stakeholders who should be involved in the risk management process. This typically includes representatives from engineering, quality assurance, regulatory affairs, clinical experts, and other relevant disciplines. Define their roles and responsibilities to ensure effective collaboration.

4. **Determine Risk Acceptability Criteria:** Establish criteria to determine the acceptability of risks associated with the medical device. These criteria may consider factors such as the severity of harm, probability of occurrence, available risk reduction measures, and applicable regulations or standards.

5. **Select Risk Management Methods and Tools:** Determine the methods and tools to be used for risk management activities. This includes selecting appropriate risk assessment techniques, such as failure mode and effects analysis (FMEA) or fault tree analysis (FTA), and identifying any specific tools or software that will be utilized.

6. **Plan Risk Management Activities:** Develop a detailed plan that outlines the specific risk management activities to be conducted. This

may include hazard identification, risk analysis, risk evaluation, risk control measures, and ongoing monitoring. Define the sequence of activities and allocate necessary resources.

7. **Document the Risk Management Plan:** Document the risk management plan in a formal document that is easily accessible to all relevant stakeholders. The plan should be clear, concise, and updated as needed throughout the device lifecycle.

8. **Review and Approval:** Review the risk management plan with key stakeholders, including management and regulatory experts, to ensure alignment with organizational goals and regulatory requirements. Obtain necessary approvals and ensure that all involved parties are aware of and committed to the plan.

Risk Management Planning lays the foundation for a structured and effective risk management process. It provides a roadmap for conducting risk management activities and ensures that the process is carried out in a systematic and consistent manner. By establishing clear objectives, defining the scope, and identifying stakeholders, the risk management plan helps ensure that risks associated with the medical device are appropriately identified, evaluated, and controlled.

3.2 RISK IDENTIFICATION

Risk Identification is a crucial step in the risk management process according to ISO 14971. It involves systematically identifying potential hazards and sources of harm associated with a medical device. Here are the key elements of the risk identification process:

1. **Establish a Risk Identification Team:** Assemble a multidisciplinary team consisting of experts from various relevant disciplines, such as engineering, design, manufacturing, quality assurance, and clinical fields. The team's diverse expertise and perspectives contribute to a comprehensive identification of potential risks.

2. **Identify Potential Hazards:** Conduct a thorough examination of the medical device, its components, and its intended use to identify potential hazards. Hazards can be physical, chemical, biological, ergonomic, or software-related. Consider all aspects, including device design, manufacturing processes, materials used, and foreseeable misuse or user errors.

3. **Utilize Information Sources:** Gather information from various sources to aid in hazard identification. These sources may include historical data, clinical studies, post-market surveillance, adverse event reports, scientific literature, and feedback from users or customers. This helps capture real-world experiences and knowledge about potential risks.

4. **Use Risk Analysis Techniques:** Employ systematic techniques to analyze the identified hazards and their potential consequences. Commonly used methods include brainstorming sessions, checklists, and structured analysis tools like fault tree analysis (FTA) or failure mode and effects analysis (FMEA). These techniques help identify potential causes and effects of hazards.

5. **Consider Foreseeable Misuse and User Errors:** Assess the likelihood of foreseeable misuse or errors by users during device operation. Analyze scenarios where users may deviate from intended use or misuse the device. This includes considering the device's user interface, labeling, instructions for use, and potential human factors issues.

6. **Document Identified Risks:** Document all identified hazards and associated risks in a systematic manner. Create a risk identification matrix or table that captures each identified hazard along with its potential consequences and associated risks. Include a description of the hazard, its potential severity of harm, and the likelihood of occurrence.

7. **Review and Validation:** Review the identified risks with the risk identification team and stakeholders to ensure completeness and accuracy. Validate the identified risks by seeking input from subject matter experts and verifying against available data sources.

8. **Maintain Traceability:** Maintain a traceable record of the identified risks throughout the risk management process. Link each risk to the subsequent steps in the process, including risk analysis, evaluation, and control measures. This ensures traceability and facilitates effective risk management.

By systematically identifying potential hazards and sources of harm, the risk identification process enables medical device manufacturers to gain a comprehensive understanding of the risks associated with their devices. It forms the basis for further risk analysis, evaluation, and the implementation of appropriate risk control measures.

3.3 RISK ANALYSIS

Risk Analysis is a critical step in the risk management process according to ISO 14971. It involves evaluating the identified risks associated with a medical device to assess their likelihood of occurrence and potential severity of harm. The key elements of the risk analysis process are as follows:

1. **Risk Estimation:** Estimate the probability or likelihood of occurrence for each identified risk. This involves analyzing available data, historical information, and expert judgment to determine the likelihood of the risk event happening. Consider factors such as device characteristics, intended use, user interactions, and external influences.

2. **Consequence Assessment:** Assess the potential severity of harm that could result from each identified risk. Evaluate the impact on patients, users, operators, and any other stakeholders. Consider both immediate and long-term consequences, including physical injury, psychological effects, and potential impact on patient outcomes.

3. **Risk Matrix:** Create a risk matrix or use a similar risk assessment tool to visualize the estimated likelihood and consequence of each risk. The risk matrix helps prioritize risks based on their potential impact. It classifies risks into different risk levels, such as low, medium, and high, based on the combination of likelihood and consequence.

4. **Risk Ranking:** Rank the identified risks based on their levels of risk, taking into account the risk matrix or assessment tool used. This helps determine the order of priority for further risk management activities. Higher-risk events with greater potential harm and likelihood should receive more attention and be addressed promptly.

5. **Risk Interactions:** Consider the interactions between different risks. Some risks may influence or exacerbate each other, leading to higher overall risk. Evaluate how the occurrence of one risk may affect the occurrence or severity of other risks. Understanding these interactions helps in developing effective risk control measures.

6. **Documentation:** Document the risk analysis process, including the estimated likelihood, consequence, risk matrix, and risk rankings. This documentation provides a clear and traceable record of the analysis performed and enables effective communication among stakeholders.

7. **Review and Validation:** Review the risk analysis results with the risk analysis team and relevant stakeholders. Validate the estimated likelihood and consequence with available data, clinical expertise, and scientific literature. Incorporate feedback and make necessary adjustments to ensure the accuracy and reliability of the risk analysis.

The risk analysis process provides a systematic and structured approach to evaluating the identified risks associated with a medical device. It helps prioritize risks based on their potential impact, facilitating effective risk management decision-making. The outcomes of the risk analysis guide subsequent steps, such as risk evaluation, risk control, and ongoing monitoring throughout the device lifecycle.

3.4 RISK EVALUATION

Risk Evaluation is a crucial step in the risk management process according to ISO 14971. It involves assessing the acceptability of identified risks associated with a medical device based on predetermined criteria. The key elements of the risk evaluation process are as follows:

1. **Establish Risk Acceptability Criteria:** Define specific criteria or thresholds for determining the acceptability of risks. These criteria can be based on regulatory requirements, industry standards, clinical guidelines, and organizational policies. Consider factors such as the severity of harm, the likelihood of occurrence, available risk reduction measures, and societal expectations.

2. **Compare Risks against Acceptability Criteria:** Compare each identified risk against the established risk acceptability criteria. Assess whether the risk level falls within acceptable limits or exceeds the predefined thresholds. This comparison helps determine whether further risk control measures are necessary or if the risks are already at an acceptable level.

3. **Consider Overall Risk Profile:** Evaluate the collective impact of all identified risks on the overall risk profile of the medical device. Take into account the cumulative effect of multiple risks and their interactions. Consider the context of the device's use, its intended population, and any specific vulnerabilities or sensitivities.

4. **Risk-Benefit Analysis:** Consider the benefits and intended purpose of the medical device in relation to the identified risks. Perform a risk-benefit analysis to assess whether the potential benefits of using the device outweigh the associated risks. This analysis helps inform risk management decisions and the determination of acceptable risk levels.

5. **Risk Reduction Measures:** Assess the effectiveness of existing risk control measures in mitigating or reducing the identified risks. Evaluate whether additional risk reduction measures are necessary to bring the risks to an acceptable level. Consider the feasibility, practicality, and impact of implementing such measures.

6. **Documentation:** Document the results of the risk evaluation process, including the determination of acceptability or unacceptability for each identified risk. Clearly record the rationale behind the decisions made, including any supporting data, expert opinions, or risk management considerations.

7. **Review and Validation:** Review the risk evaluation results with the risk management team and relevant stakeholders. Validate the conclusions reached through appropriate verification and validation activities. Incorporate feedback and make any necessary adjustments to ensure the accuracy and reliability of the risk evaluation.

The risk evaluation process ensures a systematic assessment of identified risks and their alignment with predetermined risk acceptability criteria. It provides a basis for making informed decisions regarding risk control measures and risk management strategies. By evaluating risks in relation to their acceptability, the process supports the overall goal of ensuring the safety and effectiveness of the medical device throughout its lifecycle.

3.5 RISK CONTROL

Risk Control is a critical step in the risk management process according to ISO 14971. It involves implementing measures to reduce or eliminate risks associated with a medical device to an acceptable level. The key elements of the risk control process are as follows:

1. **Identify Risk Control Options:** Identify and evaluate various risk control options available for managing the identified risks. These options can include design changes, process modifications, safety features, warnings and instructions, protective measures, training programs, and quality control measures.

2. **Hierarchy of Risk Control Measures:** Apply the principles of the hierarchy of controls to select appropriate risk control measures. The hierarchy of controls includes the following options in order of priority: elimination, substitution, engineering controls, administrative controls, and personal protective equipment (PPE). Prioritize measures that eliminate or reduce risks at the source rather than relying on protective measures alone.

3. **Implement Risk Control Measures:** Implement the selected risk control measures to reduce or eliminate the identified risks. This may involve making design changes, modifying manufacturing processes,

enhancing safety features, developing clear warnings and instructions, providing training programs for users and operators, and implementing quality control procedures.

4. **Verify Effectiveness of Risk Controls:** Verify and validate the effectiveness of the implemented risk control measures. This may involve conducting testing, simulations, and assessments to ensure that the controls adequately reduce or mitigate the identified risks. The verification process helps ensure that the implemented measures are achieving the desired risk reduction.

5. **Document Risk Control Measures:** Document the implemented risk control measures in the risk management file. Clearly describe the specific control measures, their purpose, and how they reduce or eliminate the identified risks. Maintain proper documentation to provide evidence of compliance with risk management requirements.

6. **Reassess Risk:** Reassess the risks after implementing the control measures to determine their residual levels. Evaluate whether the implemented measures have effectively reduced the risks to an acceptable level. If the residual risks are still unacceptable, additional control measures may be required.

7. **Monitor and Review:** Continuously monitor and review the effectiveness of the implemented risk control measures throughout the device's lifecycle. Regularly assess the device's performance, safety data, post-market surveillance reports, and feedback from users to identify any new risks or changes in existing risks. Update risk control measures as necessary based on the outcomes of monitoring and reviews.

8. **Post-Market Surveillance:** Establish post-market surveillance activities to detect, analyze, and address any new risks or changes in risks that emerge after the device is on the market. This includes processes for collecting and analyzing adverse events, customer feedback, and other relevant information to ensure ongoing risk management.

The risk control process aims to minimize risks associated with a medical device by implementing appropriate measures. It ensures that the identified risks are effectively addressed and reduced to an acceptable level, contributing to the safety and performance of the device throughout its lifecycle.

3.6 RISK ASSESSMENT AND RESIDUAL RISK EVALUATION

Risk Assessment and Residual Risk Evaluation are crucial steps in the risk management process according to ISO 14971. They involve the systematic evaluation of risks associated with a medical device, including both inherent risks and those that remain after implementing risk control measures. The key elements of these steps are as follows:

1. **RISK ASSESSMENT:**

    a. **Review Identified Risks:** Review the risks identified during the risk identification and analysis steps. Consider both the severity of harm and the likelihood of occurrence for each identified risk.

    b. **Evaluate Risk Factors:** Evaluate various factors that contribute to the overall risk level, such as the probability of occurrence, severity of harm, detectability, and impact on the target population or users. These factors help in assessing the significance of each risk.

    c. **Assign Risk Levels:** Assign risk levels or scores to each identified risk based on the evaluation of risk factors. This may involve using a risk matrix or other risk assessment tools to categorize risks into different levels (e.g., low, medium, high) or numerical scales.

    d. **Prioritize Risks:** Prioritize the identified risks based on their risk levels. Focus on risks with higher levels of severity or likelihood that require immediate attention. This prioritization helps in allocating resources effectively and addressing the most critical risks first.

2. **RESIDUAL RISK EVALUATION:**

    a. **Assess Effectiveness of Risk Control Measures:** Evaluate the effectiveness of the implemented risk control measures in reducing or mitigating the identified risks. Consider the residual risks that remain after implementing these measures.

b. **Reassess Risk Factors:** Reassess the risk factors for each identified risk, taking into account the impact of the implemented risk control measures. This includes considering factors such as the reduced probability of occurrence, decreased severity of harm, and improved detectability.

c. **Determine Residual Risk Levels:** Determine the residual risk levels for each identified risk after implementing the risk control measures. This involves evaluating the remaining risk factors and assigning appropriate risk levels or scores to reflect the residual risk.

d. **Compare Residual Risks with Acceptability Criteria:** Compare the residual risks against the predetermined risk acceptability criteria established in the risk evaluation step. Assess whether the residual risks fall within acceptable limits or if further actions are required to bring them to an acceptable level.

e. **Document Residual Risks:** Document the residual risks along with their assigned risk levels and any necessary actions or recommendations for further risk management. Maintain traceability by linking the residual risks to the risk control measures implemented and the risk management decisions made.

Risk Assessment and Residual Risk Evaluation ensure a comprehensive evaluation of risks associated with a medical device, both before and after implementing risk control measures. These steps help in assessing the overall risk profile of the device, prioritizing risks, and making informed decisions regarding risk management strategies. By considering the residual risks, the process ensures that the remaining risks are at an acceptable level and in compliance with regulatory requirements.

3.7 RISK MANAGEMENT REVIEW

Risk Management Review is an essential step in the risk management process according to ISO 14971. It involves systematically reviewing and evaluating the effectiveness of the risk management activities performed throughout the lifecycle of a medical device. The key elements of the risk management review process are as follows:

1. **Schedule Regular Reviews:** Establish a predetermined schedule for conducting risk management reviews at appropriate intervals throughout the device's lifecycle. These reviews should be conducted at significant milestones, such as during design and development, before regulatory submissions, and post-market surveillance.

2. **Evaluate Risk Management Process:** Assess the overall effectiveness of the risk management process implemented for the medical device. Review whether the risk management activities, such as risk identification, analysis, evaluation, and control, were conducted according to established procedures and regulatory requirements.

3. **Review Risk Management File:** Examine the risk management file, which contains documentation of all risk management activities, including risk assessments, risk control measures, and risk management decisions. Ensure that the file is complete, up-to-date, and accurately reflects the risk management process.

4. **Assess Compliance:** Evaluate the compliance of the risk management activities with applicable regulatory requirements, industry standards, and organizational policies. Determine if the risk management process followed the principles outlined in ISO 14971 and if any deviations or non-compliance issues need to be addressed.

5. **Review Risk Acceptability:** Review the acceptability of the identified risks, taking into account any changes in circumstances, new information, or updated risk acceptance criteria. Assess whether the risks are still at an acceptable level or if additional risk control measures are necessary to maintain an acceptable risk profile.

6. **Evaluate Risk Controls:** Assess the effectiveness of the implemented risk control measures in reducing or eliminating risks. Consider feedback from post-market surveillance, adverse event reports, customer feedback, and other sources of information to identify any issues or areas for improvement in risk controls.

7. **Identify Lessons Learned:** Identify and document any lessons learned from previous risk management activities. This includes capturing insights, best practices, and areas of improvement to enhance future risk management processes and decision-making.

8. **Update Risk Management Plan:** Based on the outcomes of the risk management review, update the risk management plan to reflect any changes in risk management strategies, objectives, or activities. Ensure that the plan aligns with the current understanding of the device and its associated risks.

9. **Communicate Findings and Recommendations:** Communicate the findings of the risk management review to relevant stakeholders, including management, regulatory bodies, and other relevant parties. Provide recommendations for any necessary actions, such as implementing additional risk control measures, revising labeling or instructions for use, or conducting further risk assessments.

10. **Document Review Results:** Document the results of the risk management review, including the findings, recommendations, and any actions taken due to the review. Maintain proper documentation to demonstrate compliance with regulatory requirements and to support the ongoing improvement of the risk management process.

The risk management review process ensures that the effectiveness of the risk management activities is continuously monitored and assessed. It provides an opportunity to identify areas for improvement, address emerging risks, and ensure the ongoing safety and effectiveness of the medical device throughout its lifecycle.

3.8 RISK MANAGEMENT REPORT

The Risk Management Report is a key deliverable in the risk management process according to ISO 14971. It provides a comprehensive summary of the risk management activities conducted for a medical device, including the identification, analysis, evaluation, control, and review of risks. The Risk Management Report serves as a documented record of the risk management process and its outcomes. The key elements of the Risk Management Report are as follows:

1. **Introduction:** Provide an overview of the purpose and scope of the Risk Management Report. Describe the medical device and its intended use, and outline the objectives of the risk management process.

2. **Risk Management Process Summary:** Summarize the key steps of the risk management process undertaken, including risk identification, analysis, evaluation, control measures implemented, and the outcomes of the risk management review.

3. **Risk Management Plan:** Include a summary of the Risk Management Plan, which outlines the approach, responsibilities, and timeline for the risk management activities. Describe any deviations or changes from the initial plan and provide a rationale for those changes.

4. **Risk Identification:** Document the identified hazards and potential risks associated with the medical device. Include a description of the potential harm, the potential causes of harm, and the affected users or patients.

5. **Risk Analysis:** Provide a detailed analysis of the identified risks. Describe the methodology used for risk analysis, such as the use of risk matrices, and present the results of the analysis, including the assigned risk levels or scores for each identified risk.

6. **Risk Evaluation:** Present the criteria used for risk evaluation and the acceptability thresholds established. Summarize the results of the risk evaluation, including the determination of whether each risk is acceptable or requires further risk control measures.

7. **Risk Control Measures:** Describe the risk control measures implemented to reduce or eliminate identified risks. Include a summary of the measures taken, such as design changes, safety features, warnings and instructions, training programs, or quality control measures.

8. **Residual Risk Evaluation:** Document the assessment of residual risks after implementing the risk control measures. Present the residual risk levels and compare them against the predetermined risk acceptability criteria.

9. **Risk Management Review:** Summarize the outcomes of the risk management review, including any findings, recommendations, and actions taken because of the review. Include any lessons learned and improvements made to the risk management process.

10. **Conclusion:** Provide a conclusion that summarizes the overall risk management process and its outcomes. Emphasize the effectiveness of the risk management activities in ensuring the safety and performance of the medical device.

11. **Annexes:** Include any relevant supporting documentation, such as risk assessment forms, risk matrices, verification and validation reports, post-market surveillance data, and other supplementary information.

The Risk Management Report serves as a comprehensive record of the risk management process undertaken for a medical device. It demonstrates compliance with regulatory requirements and provides evidence of the thorough evaluation and control of risks associated with the device. The report is an important document for regulatory submissions, audits, and ongoing risk management activities throughout the lifecycle of the medical device.

3.9 POST-MARKET SURVEILLANCE AND FEEDBACK

Post-market surveillance and feedback play a crucial role in the risk management process for medical devices. It involves actively monitoring the device's performance and safety once it is on the market, collecting and analyzing data from various sources, and incorporating feedback from users, healthcare professionals, and regulatory authorities. The key elements of post-market surveillance and feedback are as follows:

1. **Establish Post-Market Surveillance Plan:** Develop a comprehensive plan for post-market surveillance activities that outlines the objectives, methodologies, and timelines for data collection and analysis. This plan should align with regulatory requirements and consider the device's risk profile, intended use, and target population.

2. **Adverse Event Reporting:** Implement a robust system for collecting and analyzing adverse event reports associated with the device. Encourage users, healthcare professionals, and other relevant stakeholders to report any incidents, malfunctions, or adverse events related to the device's use.

3. **Complaint Handling:** Establish a process for handling and investigating complaints related to the device. Ensure that complaints are properly recorded, categorized, and analyzed to identify potential risks or issues requiring further action.

4. **Post-Market Clinical Follow-up:** Conduct post-market clinical follow-up studies or investigations to assess the device's performance and safety in real-world clinical settings. This may involve collecting data on patient outcomes, device-related complications, and long-term effects.

5. **Trend Analysis:** Analyze collected data to identify any emerging trends or patterns related to device performance, safety, or potential risks. Monitor changes in the frequency or severity of adverse events and complaints over time and assess their potential impact on patient safety.

6. **Periodic Safety Update Reports (PSUR):** Prepare periodic safety update reports, as required by regulatory authorities, to summarize the device's safety and performance data collected during post-market surveillance. These reports provide an overview of adverse events, complaints, and any changes in risk assessment or risk management measures.

7. **Risk Management Review:** Integrate post-market surveillance data into the risk management review process. Assess whether the identified risks remain acceptable or require any updates to risk control measures, warnings, instructions for use, or other risk management activities.

8. **Feedback Collection:** Actively seek feedback from users, healthcare professionals, and regulatory authorities regarding the device's performance, usability, and safety. This can be done through surveys, user feedback programs, clinical evaluations, and interactions with regulatory agencies.

9. **Continuous Improvement:** Use the insights gained from post-market surveillance and feedback to drive continuous improvement of the device and its risk management process. Identify opportunities for design enhancements, labeling updates, training programs, or other measures to further enhance the device's safety and performance.

10. **Regulatory Reporting:** Comply with regulatory requirements for reporting adverse events, field safety corrective actions, product recalls, and other safety-related information to regulatory authorities promptly.

Post-market surveillance and feedback provide valuable information for assessing and managing risks associated with medical devices. They help detect and address potential safety issues, support the ongoing monitoring of device performance, and contribute to the overall improvement of patient safety. By actively engaging with users and other stakeholders, manufacturers can proactively respond to feedback, address concerns, and continuously enhance the device's safety and effectiveness.

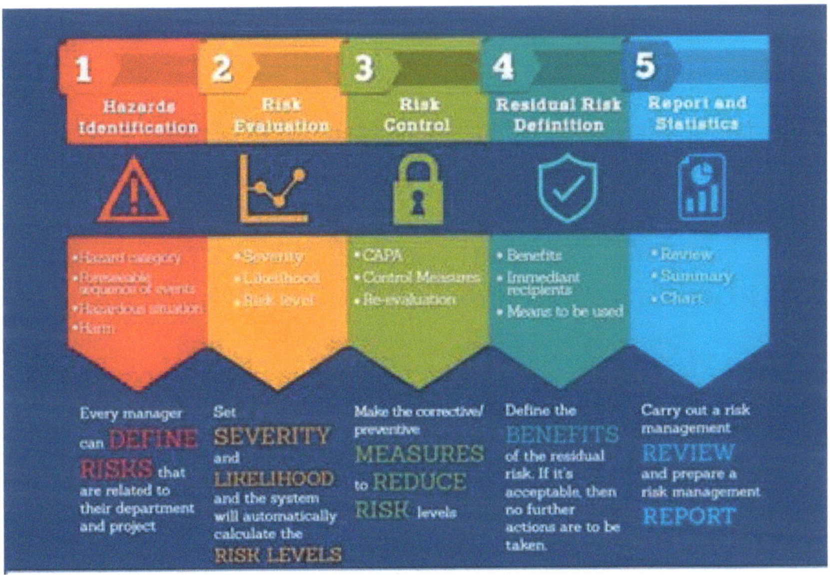

FIGURE: 3.2 RISK MANAGEMENT PROCESS ACCORDING TO ISO 14971

CHAPTER-4

RISK MANAGEMENT TOOLS AND TECHNIQUES

Risk management in the medical device industry involves the use of various tools and techniques to identify, assess, control, and monitor risks systematically. These tools and techniques aid in making informed decisions and implementing effective risk mitigation strategies. Here are some commonly used risk management tools and techniques:

1. **Risk Assessment Matrix:** A risk assessment matrix, also known as a risk matrix, is a visual tool that helps in assessing the severity of harm and the probability of occurrence for identified risks. It categorizes risks into different risk levels based on predefined criteria, such as low, medium, and high. This tool enables prioritization of risks and facilitates decision-making regarding risk control measures.

2. **Failure Mode and Effects Analysis (FMEA):** FMEA is a systematic technique (Figure 4.1) used to identify potential failure modes in a device, determine their causes and effects, and evaluate their severity, occurrence, and detectability. It helps in proactively identifying and mitigating risks by assessing the likelihood of failures and their potential impact on patient safety.

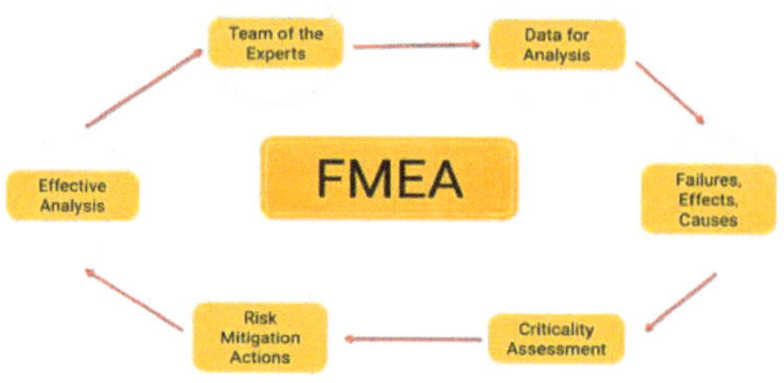

FIGURE 4.1: OVERVIEW OF FMEA

3. **Fault Tree Analysis (FTA):** FTA is a graphical technique used to analyze the logical relationships between failures and their contributing factors. It helps in understanding how different events or failures can lead to a specific undesired outcome. FTA assists in identifying critical events or failures that can lead to severe consequences and guides the development of risk control measures.

4. **Hazard Analysis and Critical Control Points (HACCP):** HACCP is a risk management approach commonly used in the food and healthcare industries. It involves identifying and controlling hazards that can affect product safety. HACCP focuses on analyzing the entire process and implementing preventive measures at critical control points to eliminate or reduce risks.

5. **Risk Control Measures:** Various risk control measures can be employed to mitigate identified risks. These measures include design modifications, safety features, protective barriers, warning labels, instructions for use, quality control procedures, training programs, and the implementation of safety guidelines and standards.

6. **Statistical Analysis:** Statistical analysis techniques, such as trend analysis, data mining, and statistical process control, can be utilized to identify patterns, trends, and anomalies in collected data. These techniques help in detecting potential risks, evaluating their significance, and making data-driven decisions.

7. **Human Factors Analysis:** Human factors analysis examines how users interact with a medical device and assesses the potential risks associated with human errors or usability issues. Techniques such as usability testing, cognitive walkthroughs, and task analysis help in identifying and addressing user-related risks.

8. **Post-Market Surveillance:** Post-market surveillance activities, including adverse event reporting, complaint handling, and data analysis, provide valuable insights into the performance and safety of a medical device in real-world scenarios. These activities help in identifying potential risks and assessing the effectiveness of risk control measures implemented.

9. **Lessons Learned and Best Practices:** Learning from past experiences and industry best practices is an essential tool for risk management.

Analyzing previous incidents, conducting root cause analysis, and sharing knowledge within the organization and with industry peers contribute to continuous improvement in risk management practices.

10. **Risk Management Software:** Risk management software tools provide a centralized platform for documenting and managing risks throughout the device lifecycle. These tools facilitate risk assessment, control measure tracking, reporting, and collaboration among stakeholders.

These tools and techniques can be employed individually or in combination, depending on the specific needs of the risk management process. Their effective utilization enhances the ability to identify, assess, control, and monitor risks associated with medical devices, ultimately improving patient safety and product quality.

4.1 HAZARD IDENTIFICATION TECHNIQUES

Hazard identification is a critical step in the risk management process. It involves systematically identifying potential hazards or sources of harm that could lead to adverse events or unsafe conditions associated with a medical device. Several techniques can be used to facilitate hazard identification. Here are some commonly employed techniques as discussed in Figure 4.2:

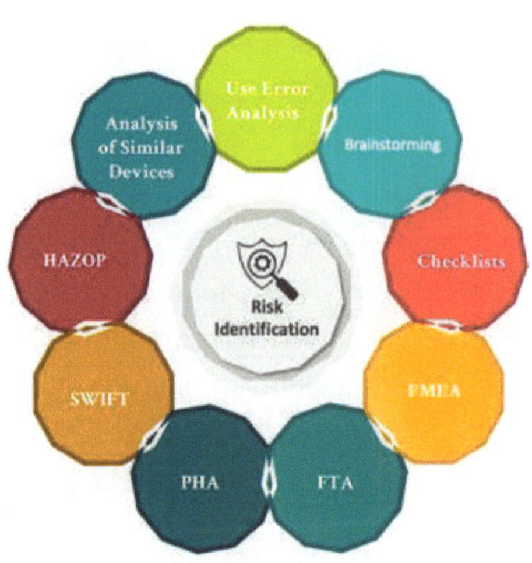

FIGURE 4.2: HAZARD IDENTIFICATION

1. **Brainstorming:** Brainstorming involves a group discussion or session where participants generate ideas and identify potential hazards related to the device. This technique encourages creative thinking and allows for a wide range of perspectives to be considered.

2. **Checklists:** Checklists are structured lists of potential hazards or risk factors specific to the medical device industry. They serve as prompts to systematically review the device's components, materials, design, manufacturing processes, and intended use to identify potential hazards.

3. **Failure Mode and Effects Analysis (FMEA):** FMEA, mentioned earlier as a risk management tool, is also used for hazard identification. It systematically analyzes each component or process step of a medical device to identify potential failure modes and their effects on the device's functionality and safety.

4. **Fault Tree Analysis (FTA):** FTA, another technique mentioned earlier, can be used for hazard identification as well. It starts with identifying the undesired outcomes or hazards and then traces back the logical pathways of failures that could lead to those outcomes.

5. **Preliminary Hazard Analysis (PHA):** PHA is an early-stage hazard identification technique that involves reviewing the device's design, specifications, and intended use to identify potential hazards and their causes. It is typically performed during the design phase to guide risk management activities.

6. **Structured What-If Technique (SWIFT):** SWIFT is a structured brainstorming technique that guides participants through a series of "what-if" questions to identify potential hazards and their causes. It encourages systematic exploration of different scenarios and their associated risks.

7. **Hazard and Operability Study (HAZOP):** HAZOP is a technique commonly used in process industries, but it can also be adapted for hazard identification in medical devices. It involves systematically

examining each element of the device or the device's processes to identify deviations from intended operation and potential hazards.

8. **Expert Panels and Reviews:** Assembling a panel of subject matter experts or conducting expert reviews can provide valuable insights into potential hazards. Experts from various domains, such as engineering, medicine, human factors, and regulatory affairs, can contribute their expertise to identify hazards associated with the device.

9. **Analysis of Similar Devices:** Analyzing similar existing devices or products can help identify potential hazards and associated risks that might be applicable to the device being assessed. It involves reviewing literature, post-market surveillance data, adverse event reports, and other sources of information to identify hazards encountered in similar devices.

10. **Use Error Analysis:** Use error analysis focuses on identifying hazards associated with human interactions with the device. It involves examining how users might misuse or misinterpret the device, leading to potential harm. Techniques such as task analysis, human factors analysis, and user feedback can assist in identifying use-related hazards.

It is important to note that hazard identification techniques are not mutually exclusive, and a combination of multiple techniques may be used to ensure comprehensive hazard identification. The choice of techniques depends on the specific device, its complexity, and the expertise available within the organization. The identified hazards serve as the foundation for further risk analysis, evaluation, and control activities within the risk management process.

4.2 RISK ANALYSIS METHODS

Risk analysis is a crucial step in the risk management process, aimed at evaluating the identified hazards and assessing their associated risks. It involves analyzing the likelihood and severity of harm resulting from the identified hazards. Several methods can be used for risk analysis in the medical device industry. Here are some commonly employed risk analysis methods (Figure 4.3):

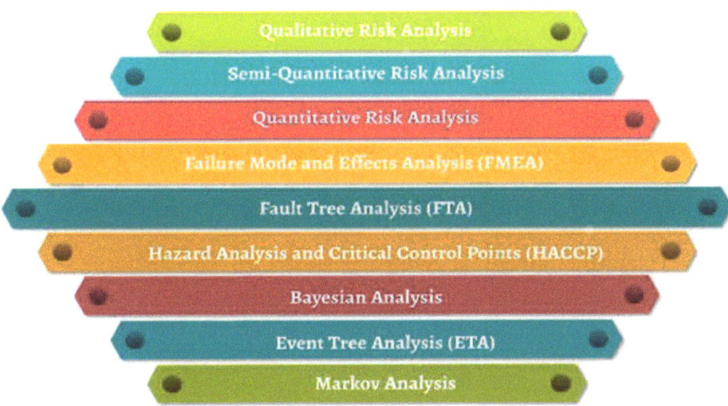

FIGURE 4.3: RISK ANALYSIS METHODS

1. **Qualitative Risk Analysis:** Qualitative risk analysis involves a subjective assessment of the likelihood and severity of harm associated with identified risks. It utilizes descriptive scales or risk matrices to categorize risks into predefined levels, such as low, medium, and high. This method is valuable for prioritizing risks based on their perceived significance without quantifying exact probabilities.

2. **Semi-Quantitative Risk Analysis:** Semi-quantitative risk analysis combines qualitative assessments with limited quantitative data. It involves assigning scores or values to the likelihood and severity of harm and multiplying them to determine a risk score. The risk scores can be categorized into risk levels or ranges, allowing for a more refined assessment of risks compared to qualitative analysis alone.

3. **Quantitative Risk Analysis:** Quantitative risk analysis involves the use of numerical data and statistical techniques to quantify the likelihood and severity of harm. It utilizes probability distributions, data modeling, and statistical analysis to calculate probabilities, frequencies, and expected consequences. This method provides a more precise and objective assessment of risks based on available data.

4. **Fault Tree Analysis (FTA):** FTA, mentioned earlier as a hazard identification technique, can also be used for risk analysis. It uses a logical and graphical representation of events and failures to assess

the probability of a specific undesired outcome. FTA quantifies the likelihood of failure events using probability values and calculates the overall probability of the undesired outcome.

5. **Failure Mode and Effects Analysis (FMEA):** FMEA, also mentioned earlier as a hazard identification technique, can be used for risk analysis as well. It involves assessing the severity, occurrence, and detectability of potential failure modes and their effects. The combination of these factors results in a risk priority number (RPN), which ranks the risks based on their potential impact.

6. **Hazard Analysis and Critical Control Points (HACCP):** HACCP, primarily used in the food and healthcare industries, can be adapted for risk analysis in medical devices. It involves identifying hazards, determining their likelihood and severity, and establishing critical control points to mitigate the risks. HACCP uses decision trees or matrices to assess risks and determine appropriate control measures.

7. **Bayesian Analysis:** Bayesian analysis combines prior knowledge or assumptions with new data to update the probabilities of risks. It incorporates subjective and objective information to estimate the likelihood and consequences of risks. Bayesian analysis is particularly useful when new data becomes available during the lifecycle of a medical device.

8. **Event Tree Analysis (ETA):** ETA is a graphical method that analyzes the consequences of a specific initiating event or hazard. It evaluates the various potential outcomes and their probabilities, allowing for a systematic assessment of risks associated with a specific event.

9. **Markov Analysis:** Markov analysis models the transition of a system between different states over time. It can be used to assess the probabilities and consequences of different states, including hazardous conditions or failures, and evaluate the associated risks.

The choice of risk analysis method depends on the available data, the complexity of the device and its use, and the desired level of detail and precision. Often, a combination of methods may be used to provide a comprehensive assessment of risks. The outcomes of risk analysis guide further risk evaluation, control measure selection, and decision-making in the risk management process.

4.3 RISK EVALUATION AND RISK ACCEPTANCE CRITERIA

Risk evaluation is a crucial step in the risk management process, where the assessed risks are compared against predefined risk acceptance criteria to determine their acceptability. Risk acceptance criteria define the threshold for acceptable risk levels based on factors such as patient safety, regulatory requirements, and organizational policies. The purpose of risk evaluation is to make informed decisions about the tolerability of risks and the need for risk control measures. Here are key aspects of risk evaluation and risk acceptance criteria:

1. **Risk Severity:** Risk severity refers to the potential impact or harm resulting from a risk if it occurs. It is assessed based on factors such as the severity of the potential injury or damage to the patient, the likelihood of the risk occurring, and the duration and reversibility of the harm. Risk severity is typically categorized into predefined levels, such as minor, moderate, serious, or critical.

2. **Risk Likelihood:** Risk likelihood assesses the probability or frequency of a risk occurring. It considers factors such as the frequency of exposure to the risk, the reliability of risk control measures, and the potential causes or contributing factors that may increase or decrease the likelihood of the risk. Likelihood is often categorized into levels such as rare, unlikely, possible, likely, or frequent.

3. **Risk Matrix:** A risk matrix is a graphical representation of the relationship It combines the severity and likelihood assessments to assign a risk level or score to each identified risk. The risk matrix helps visualize the overall risk profile and aids in prioritizing risks for further action based on their combination of severity and likelihood. Table 4.1 and Figure 4.4 depicts the Accessibility of risk and their different zones.

Red Zone	Unacceptable	Cannot be accepted, however if risk control measures lead to either AFAP or Broadly acceptable, then risk is acceptable
Yellow Zone	As far as possible (AFAP)	The risk reduced to as far as possible, however, if risk control measures further can ensure keeping the same level over a period of time with further investigation into the existence of risk, then risk may be considered to be acceptable, being as far as possible. The risk is Acceptable with continuous monitoring of the residual risk through PMS Activities
Green Zone	Broadly Acceptable	The risk has been reduced to as far as possible

TABLE 4.1. ACCEPTABILITY OF RISK

Probability	5					
	4					
	3					
	2					
	1					
		1	2	3	4	5
				Severity		

	Broadly Accepted
	AFAP (As far as possible)
	Not accepted

FIGURE 4.4. DIFFERENT ZONES FOR ACCEPTABILITY OF THE RISK

4. **Risk Acceptance Criteria:** Risk acceptance criteria define the thresholds or limits for acceptable risks based on the organization's risk tolerance, regulatory requirements, and other factors. These criteria may be predefined by regulatory agencies, industry standards, or internal policies. They help determine whether a risk is acceptable or requires further risk control measures.

5. **AFAP Principle:** AFAP stands for "as far as possible." It is a principle used in risk evaluation to assess whether the risks associated with a medical device are reduced to a level that is reasonably achievable and acceptable. The AFAP principle considers the balance between the potential benefits of the device and the risks associated with its use.

6. **Risk-Benefit Analysis:** Risk evaluation involves considering the potential benefits of the medical device in relation to its associated risks. Risk-benefit analysis weighs the anticipated benefits, such as improved patient outcomes or quality of life, against the identified risks to determine whether the benefits outweigh the risks and justify the use of the device.

7. **Risk Decision Criteria:** Risk decision criteria provide guidance on the actions to be taken based on the evaluated risks. These criteria may include specific instructions or thresholds for risk acceptance, risk mitigation, or further investigation. They help ensure consistency and objectivity in decision-making regarding risk management.

The risk evaluation process involves comparing the assessed risks against the risk acceptance criteria and making informed decisions based on the outcomes. If a risk exceeds the predefined acceptance criteria, further risk control measures should be implemented to reduce the risk to an acceptable level. On the other hand, risks that fall within the acceptable criteria may be deemed tolerable without the need for additional control measures, although ongoing monitoring and reassessment may still be necessary.

It is important to note that risk acceptance criteria may vary depending on factors such as the device's intended use, its classification, the target population, and regulatory requirements in different regions. Organizations should establish their risk acceptance criteria in alignment with applicable regulations and standards, considering the specific context of their medical device and the needs of the patients and users.

4.4 RISK CONTROL STRATEGIES

Risk control strategies, also known as risk mitigation strategies, are measures implemented to reduce the identified risks to an acceptable level. These strategies aim to minimize the likelihood of harm or the severity of its consequences. When developing risk control strategies, it is important to consider the hierarchy of controls, which prioritizes the most effective and reliable approaches. Here are common risk control strategies used in the medical device industry (Figure 4.5):

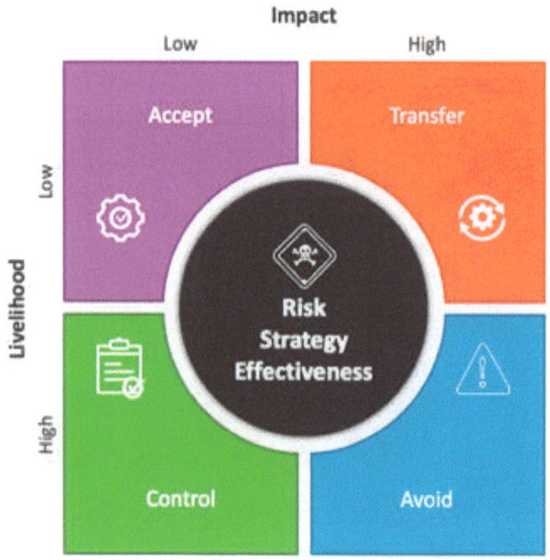

FIGURE 4.5: STRATEGIES

1. **Elimination or Removal of the Hazard:** The most effective strategy is to eliminate or remove the hazard altogether. This can be achieved by redesigning the device, modifying the manufacturing process, or removing a component or feature that poses a risk. By eliminating the hazard, the associated risk is completely eradicated.

2. **Substitution:** Substitution involves replacing a hazardous component, material, or process with a safer alternative. This strategy aims to reduce the risk by using a less hazardous option. For example, substituting a toxic material with a non-toxic one or replacing a complex component with a simpler and more reliable one.

3. **Engineering Controls:** Engineering controls involve designing and implementing safety features or protective mechanisms to minimize the risk of harm. These controls are built into the device itself or its environment to reduce the likelihood or severity of hazards. Examples include safety interlocks, physical barriers, fail-safe mechanisms, and ergonomic designs.

4. **Administrative Controls:** Administrative controls focus on implementing policies, procedures, and practices to manage and mitigate risks. These controls include guidelines for device use, training programs for users and healthcare professionals, standard operating procedures, and safety protocols. Administrative controls aim to promote safe practices and reduce human errors that may contribute to risks.

5. **Warning Labels and Instructions:** Proper labeling and clear instructions for device use are essential risk control measures. Warning labels provide information about potential hazards, precautions, and instructions for safe use. Instructions for use (IFUs) provide detailed guidance on proper device operation, maintenance, and troubleshooting. Effective communication through labeling and instructions helps users understand and mitigate risks associated with the device.

6. **Protective Equipment and Personal Protective Equipment (PPE):** In some cases, the use of protective equipment or PPE can reduce the risk of harm. This strategy involves providing users with protective gear, such as gloves, masks, goggles, or shields, to minimize exposure to hazards. PPE should be appropriate for the specific risks associated with the device and its intended use.

7. **Risk Reduction through Redundancy:** Redundancy refers to incorporating backup or duplicate systems or components to minimize

the impact of a failure or hazard. This strategy can increase the reliability and resilience of the device by providing alternative pathways or backup mechanisms to ensure safe operation in case of a failure.

8. **Maintenance and Inspection:** Regular maintenance and inspection protocols help identify and address potential risks associated with device wear and tear, component degradation, or malfunctions. Scheduled maintenance activities, including calibration, cleaning, and equipment checks, contribute to risk control by ensuring the device remains in optimal working condition.

9. **Post-Market Surveillance and Feedback:** Continuous monitoring of post-market data, including adverse event reports, complaints, and feedback from users and healthcare professionals, helps identify emerging risks and implement appropriate risk control measures. Timely action based on post-market surveillance data contributes to ongoing risk management and improvement of device safety.

10. **User Training and Education:** Adequate user training and education play a vital role in risk control. Providing comprehensive training programs and educational materials to users and healthcare professionals ensures they understand the device's proper use, limitations, and potential risks. Well-informed users are more likely to use the device safely and take appropriate measures to mitigate risks.

It is important to note that risk control strategies should be selected based on the specific risks identified during the risk management process. The combination of multiple strategies may be necessary to address different aspects of risk. The effectiveness of the chosen strategies should be evaluated and validated to ensure they adequately mitigate the identified risks and contribute to the overall safety of the medical device.

4.5 RISK MITIGATION MEASURES

Risk mitigation measures are specific actions or interventions implemented to reduce the identified risks associated with a medical device. These measures aim to minimize the likelihood and severity of harm to patients, users, and others affected by the device. Here are some common risk mitigation measures used in the medical device industry (Figure 4.6):

1. **Design Modifications:** Modifying the design of the device to eliminate or minimize the hazards is a primary risk mitigation measure. This may involve changing the materials, components, or structure of the device to improve safety and reduce the potential for harm.

2. **Enhancing Safety Features:** Adding or improving safety features can mitigate risks associated with device use. Examples include incorporating safety interlocks, alarms, fail-safe mechanisms, and protective barriers to prevent or mitigate potential hazards.

3. **Improving Manufacturing Processes:** Enhancing manufacturing processes can help reduce risks associated with device quality and performance. Implementing stricter quality control measures, conducting thorough inspections, and ensuring adherence to manufacturing standards can minimize the occurrence of defects or failures.

4. **Implementing Controls and Alarms:** Installing controls and alarms can help users and healthcare professionals monitor and manage risks. These may include visual indicators, auditory alarms, pressure limits, temperature controls, or other monitoring systems that alert users to potential hazards or abnormal conditions.

5. **Providing Training and Education:** Offering comprehensive training programs and educational materials to users, healthcare professionals, and maintenance personnel is a critical risk mitigation measure. Proper training ensures that individuals understand the device's correct operation, maintenance requirements, and potential risks. Well-trained users are more likely to use the device safely and take appropriate measures to mitigate risks.

6. **Establishing Standard Operating Procedures (SOPs):** Developing and implementing SOPs provides clear guidelines for device use, maintenance, and troubleshooting. SOPs help ensure consistent and

safe practices by outlining step-by-step procedures and precautions to be followed during various device-related activities.

7. **Conducting Clinical Trials and Studies:** Clinical trials and studies provide an opportunity to assess the safety and effectiveness of a medical device in a controlled environment. By collecting data on device performance and adverse events, these trials can help identify potential risks and inform risk mitigation strategies before widespread use.

8. **Labeling and Instructions for Use:** Clear and comprehensive labeling, including warnings, precautions, contraindications, and instructions for use, is a crucial risk mitigation measure. Properly labeled devices provide essential information to users and healthcare professionals, enabling them to understand and mitigate risks associated with device use.

9. **Implementing Quality Management Systems (QMS):** Establishing robust QMS, such as complying with ISO 13485, helps ensure effective risk management throughout the device's lifecycle. QMS provides a framework for identifying, assessing, and mitigating risks, as well as monitoring and documenting risk-related activities.

10. **Post-Market Surveillance and Vigilance:** Implementing post-market surveillance activities, such as monitoring adverse events, complaints, and user feedback, allows for the identification of potential risks associated with the device's real-world use. Timely collection and analysis of post-market data enable proactive risk mitigation and continuous improvement of device safety.

11. **Establishing Feedback Mechanisms:** Providing channels for users, healthcare professionals, and other stakeholders to report concerns, suggestions, and adverse events is essential for risk mitigation. Feedback mechanisms enable the timely identification and resolution of device-related risks and contribute to ongoing improvement efforts.

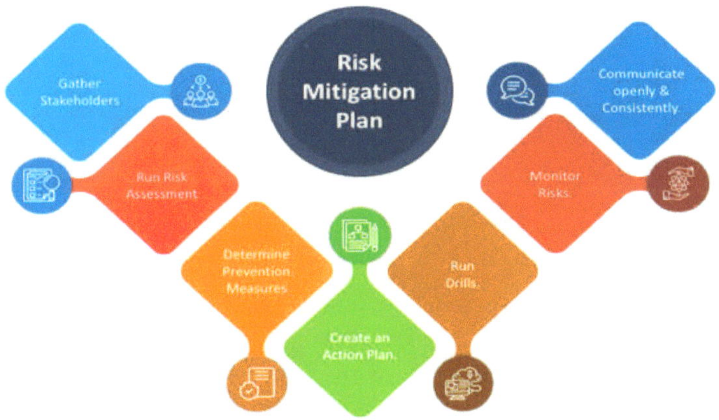

FIGURE 4.6: RISK MITIGATION PLAN

It is important to note that risk mitigation measures should be tailored to the specific risks identified during the risk management process. The effectiveness of these measures should be evaluated and validated to ensure they adequately mitigate the identified risks and contribute to the overall safety of the medical device.

4.6 RISK COMMUNICATION AND DOCUMENTATION

Risk communication (as summarized by Figure 4.7) and documentation are essential components of the risk management process in the medical device industry. Effective communication ensures that relevant stakeholders, including regulatory authorities, healthcare professionals, users, and patients, are informed about the identified risks, risk mitigation measures, and any necessary actions. Documentation provides a record of the risk management activities undertaken, facilitating traceability, accountability, and regulatory compliance. Here are key aspects of risk communication and documentation:

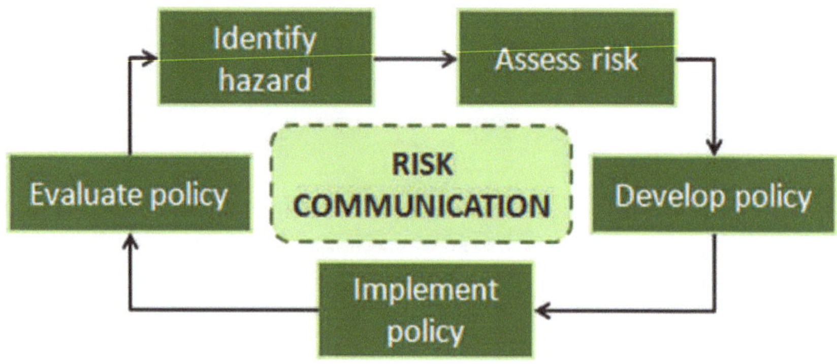

Figure 4.7 : Risk Communication Process Chart

1. **Risk Communication:**

   - **Stakeholder Engagement:** Engaging relevant stakeholders throughout the risk management process fosters transparency and collaboration. Stakeholders may include regulatory agencies, healthcare professionals, users, patient advocacy groups, and internal organizational members.

   - **Clear and Concise Messaging:** Risk information should be communicated in a clear and understandable manner, avoiding technical jargon. It should address the potential risks, their implications, and recommended actions, while also considering the target audience's level of knowledge and expertise.

   - **Timeliness:** Risk communication should occur on time, ensuring that stakeholders receive the necessary information promptly to make informed decisions. This includes timely reporting of adverse events, safety concerns, and updates on risk mitigation measures.

   - **Multiple Communication Channels:** Utilizing multiple communication channels, such as product labeling, instructional materials, websites, newsletters, and direct notifications, helps reach a broader audience and ensures the dissemination of relevant risk-related information.

   - **Compliance with Regulatory Requirements:** Compliance with regulatory requirements for risk communication, including reporting obligations, labeling requirements, and post-market surveillance activities, is crucial. Adhering to these requirements ensures alignment with regulatory expectations and facilitates timely and accurate communication.

2. **Risk Documentation:**

- **Risk Management Plan (RMP):** The RMP outlines the overall risk management approach for the medical device. It provides a comprehensive overview of the risk management process, including risk identification, analysis, evaluation, control measures, and ongoing monitoring.

- **Risk Assessment Reports:** These reports document the outcomes of risk identification, analysis, and evaluation activities. They provide detailed information about the identified risks, their severity, likelihood, and risk levels, as well as supporting data and rationale.

- **Risk Control Measures:** Documentation should capture the risk control measures implemented to mitigate identified risks. This includes details about design modifications, safety features, labeling changes, manufacturing process improvements, and other measures taken to reduce risks.

- **Post-Market Surveillance Reports:** These reports summarize the findings from post-market surveillance activities, such as adverse event monitoring, complaint analysis, and user feedback. They document any newly identified risks, updates on existing risks, and actions taken to address them.

- **Standard Operating Procedures (SOPs):** SOPs related to risk management activities should be documented, providing step-by-step instructions on conducting risk assessments, implementing risk control measures, and monitoring risk throughout the device's lifecycle.

- **Change Control Documentation:** Any changes made to the device design, manufacturing processes, labeling, or risk control measures should be documented through a change control process. This ensures that the impact of changes on risk management is assessed and appropriate actions are taken.

- **Training Records:** Documentation of training programs and records of individuals who have received training on risk management processes and procedures help demonstrate compliance and competency in managing risks.

Proper risk communication and documentation facilitate knowledge sharing, regulatory compliance, and the continuous improvement of risk management practices. They contribute to the overall effectiveness of risk management efforts in ensuring the safety and performance of medical devices.

CHAPTER-5

INTEGRATION OF RISK MANAGEMENT INTO THE PRODUCT LIFE CYCLE

Integrating risk management into the product life cycle (Figure 5.1) is crucial for ensuring the safety and effectiveness of medical devices from concept to post-market surveillance. By incorporating risk management activities at each stage of the product life cycle, potential risks can be identified, assessed, and mitigated early on, leading to safer products and improved patient outcomes. Here's an overview of how risk management can be integrated into different stages of the product life cycle:

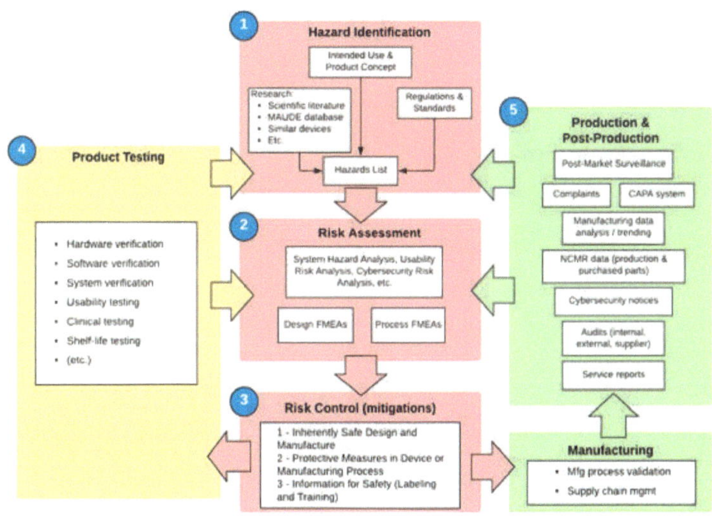

FIGURE 5.1: RISK MANAGEMENT ACROSS THE PRODUCT LIFE CYCLE

1. **CONCEPT AND PLANNING PHASE:**

   - **Identify Potential Hazards:** During the concept and planning phase, potential hazards associated with the medical device and its intended use should be identified. This includes considering the device's design, materials, technologies, and intended user population.

   - **Conduct Preliminary Risk Assessment:** Perform an initial risk assessment to identify and evaluate potential risks. This assessment helps inform the development of risk management plans and guides subsequent development activities.

2. **DESIGN AND DEVELOPMENT PHASE:**

   - **Detailed Risk Analysis:** Perform a comprehensive risk analysis to identify and evaluate risks associated with the device's design, components, manufacturing processes, and intended use. Use techniques such as FMEA (Failure Mode and Effects Analysis) and FTA (Fault Tree Analysis) to systematically assess potential failures and their consequences.

   - **Risk Control Measures:** Implement risk control measures to mitigate identified risks. This may involve design modifications, safety features, manufacturing process improvements, or other strategies to reduce risks to acceptable levels.

   - **Verification and Validation:** Verify and validate the effectiveness of risk control measures through testing, simulations, and clinical evaluations. This ensures that the implemented measures adequately mitigate identified risks and meet performance requirements.

3. **PRODUCTION AND MANUFACTURING PHASE:**

   - **Quality Management Systems:** Establish and maintain robust quality management systems (QMS) to ensure consistent production and adherence to risk management principles. This includes implementing procedures for equipment calibration, process validation, and inspection to minimize the risk of manufacturing defects.

- **Supplier Controls:** Implement supplier evaluation and control processes to assess the risks associated with outsourced components, materials, or services. This ensures that suppliers meet quality and safety requirements and helps mitigate supply chain risks.

4. **MARKETING AND COMMERCIALIZATION PHASE:**

- **Labeling and Instructions for Use:** Develop clear and comprehensive labeling and instructions for use (IFUs) that communicate potential risks, proper device usage, and necessary precautions to users, healthcare professionals, and patients.

- **Post-Market Surveillance Planning:** Develop a post-market surveillance plan to monitor the device's real-world performance, including the collection and analysis of adverse event reports, complaints, and other relevant data. This allows for the identification of emerging risks and facilitates timely risk mitigation actions.

5. **POST-MARKET PHASE:**

- **Post-Market Surveillance:** Continuously monitor and evaluate the device's performance and safety in real-world settings through post-market surveillance activities. This includes analyzing adverse events, conducting trend analysis, and collecting feedback from users and healthcare professionals to identify and address any new or recurring risks.

- **Risk Communication and Reporting:** Maintain effective communication channels to inform regulatory authorities promptly, healthcare professionals, and users about identified risks, safety concerns, and any necessary actions. This includes complying with regulatory reporting requirements for adverse events, field safety corrective actions, and updates to labeling or instructions for use.

Integrating risk management into the product life cycle ensures that risks are systematically addressed and managed throughout the device's entire lifecycle. This approach promotes the development of safe and effective medical devices, enhances patient safety, and supports regulatory compliance.

5.1 RISK MANAGEMENT DURING PRODUCT DEVELOPMENT

Risk management during product development is a critical phase in the lifecycle of a medical device. It involves identifying, analyzing, and mitigating potential risks associated with the device's design, development, and manufacturing processes. By proactively addressing risks during this phase, potential hazards can be minimized, and the overall safety and performance of the device can be enhanced. Here are key aspects of risk management during product development:

1. **Risk Identification:**

    - **Identify Potential Hazards:** Thoroughly analyze the device's intended use, design, materials, and technologies to identify potential hazards that may pose risks to users, patients, or other stakeholders.

    - **Consider Use Scenarios:** Evaluate the device's intended use scenarios, including normal use, foreseeable misuse, and off-label use, to identify potential risks and associated harm.

2. **Risk Assessment:**

    - **Risk Analysis:** Systematically analyze identified hazards to assess their potential severity, likelihood of occurrence, and detectability. Use risk analysis techniques such as FMEA (Failure Mode and Effects Analysis) and FTA (Fault Tree Analysis) to evaluate possible failure modes and their consequences.

    - **Risk Evaluation:** Evaluate the identified risks based on their severity and probability to determine their overall risk levels. This helps prioritize risks for further mitigation efforts.

3. **Risk Control:**

    - **Implement Risk Control Measures:** Develop and implement risk control measures to mitigate identified risks. These measures may include design modifications, safety features, process improvements, or warnings and precautions in the device's labeling and instructions for use.

- **Design Validation and Verification:** Validate and verify the effectiveness of risk control measures through testing, simulations, and other validation activities. This ensures that the implemented measures adequately mitigate identified risks and meet performance requirements.

4. **Design and Process Validation:**

   - **Design Validation:** Validate the design of the medical device to ensure that it meets the intended use requirements, functional specifications, and performance criteria. This includes conducting design reviews, usability testing, and clinical evaluations.

   - **Process Validation:** Validate the manufacturing processes to ensure that they consistently produce devices that meet the design specifications. This may involve process qualification, process monitoring, and statistical analysis to ensure process control and minimize the risk of manufacturing defects.

5. **Documentation and Traceability:**

   - **Maintain Documentation:** Document all risk management activities, including risk assessments, risk control measures, design validations, and process validations. This documentation provides a traceable record of the risk management process and demonstrates compliance with regulatory requirements.

   - **Risk Management File:** Compile all relevant risk management documentation into a Risk Management File, which serves as a comprehensive record of the device's risk management activities throughout the product development phase.

6. **Collaboration and Communication:**

   - **Cross-Functional Collaboration:** Foster collaboration among multidisciplinary teams, including engineers, designers, clinicians, regulatory experts, and quality professionals. This facilitates the sharing of knowledge and expertise to identify, assess, and mitigate risks effectively.

- **Communication with Stakeholders:** Maintain open and transparent communication with stakeholders, including regulatory authorities, to address any concerns, provide updates on risk management activities, and ensure alignment with regulatory requirements.

By incorporating risk management into the product development phase, manufacturers can identify and address potential risks early in the device's lifecycle. This proactive approach promotes the development of safe and effective medical devices while minimizing the potential for harm to users and patients. It also supports regulatory compliance and fosters confidence in the device's safety and performance.

5.2 RISK MANAGEMENT DURING MANUFACTURING

Risk management during the manufacturing phase of medical devices is crucial for ensuring consistent quality, compliance with regulatory requirements, and the safety and performance of the devices. This phase involves implementing processes and controls to mitigate risks associated with manufacturing operations, supply chain management, and product quality. Here are key aspects of risk management during manufacturing:

1. **Process Validation:**
   - **Establish Process Controls:** Implement robust process controls to ensure consistent manufacturing operations and minimize the risk of defects or variations in the device's quality or performance.
   - **Process Qualification:** Validate manufacturing processes to demonstrate their capability to consistently produce devices that meet the design specifications. This involves conducting process qualification studies, including process performance qualification (PPQ) and process validation activities.
   - **Statistical Process Control (SPC):** Use SPC techniques to monitor and control key process parameters during manufacturing. This helps identify process variations and ensures that the manufacturing processes remain within the specified control limits.

2. **Supplier Controls:**

   - **Supplier Qualification:** Implement a robust supplier qualification process to assess and select suppliers based on their ability to meet quality and regulatory requirements. This includes evaluating their quality management systems, capabilities, and track record.

   - **Supplier Audits and Monitoring:** Conduct periodic audits and assessments of suppliers to ensure ongoing compliance with quality and regulatory requirements. Establish clear criteria for accepting or rejecting incoming materials or components based on predefined quality standards.

   - **Supplier Corrective Actions:** Implement processes to address and resolve quality issues or non-conformities identified with suppliers. This includes initiating corrective and preventive actions (CAPA) and working collaboratively with suppliers to rectify the issues.

3. **Change Control:**

   - **Change Management Process:** Establish a change control process to evaluate and manage any changes to the manufacturing processes, materials, or components. This includes assessing the impact of changes on device quality, safety, and regulatory compliance, and ensuring appropriate risk mitigation measures are implemented.

   - **Risk Assessment for Changes:** Perform risk assessments for proposed changes to identify potential risks and evaluate their impact on device safety and performance. This helps determine the level of scrutiny and verification/validation activities needed for the change.

4. **Quality Management Systems:**

   - **Documentation and Record keeping:** Maintain accurate and comprehensive documentation of manufacturing processes, procedures, work instructions, and records of production activities. This ensures traceability and provides evidence of compliance with quality and regulatory requirements.

- **Non-Conformance Management:** Establish procedures for handling non-conforming products or processes. This includes documenting and investigating non-conformities, implementing corrective and preventive actions, and monitoring their effectiveness.

- **Internal Audits:** Conduct regular internal audits of manufacturing processes and quality systems to ensure compliance with applicable standards and regulations. These audits help identify areas for improvement and ensure ongoing adherence to established procedures.

5. **Risk-based Inspections and Testing:**

   - **Risk-based Sampling:** Develop risk-based sampling plans to determine the frequency and extent of inspections and testing during manufacturing. This ensures that critical quality parameters are adequately monitored and controlled.

   - **In-process Inspections:** Implement in-process inspections to verify the quality and conformity of the device during various stages of manufacturing. This includes visual inspections, measurements, and functional testing as necessary.

   - **Finished Product Testing:** Conduct final product testing to confirm that the device meets all specified requirements, including safety, performance, and regulatory compliance.

6. **Post-Market Surveillance:**

   - **Feedback and Complaint Handling:** Establish processes for capturing, investigating, and addressing post-market feedback, complaints, and adverse events related to the manufactured devices. This helps identify any potential risks or quality issues and facilitates timely corrective actions.

By implementing robust risk management practices during manufacturing, medical device manufacturers can ensure consistent product quality, compliance with regulatory requirements, and patient safety. This approach helps identify and mitigate manufacturing-related risks, maintain process control, and continuously improve manufacturing operations.

5.3 RISK MANAGEMENT DURING DISTRIBUTION AND SUPPLY CHAIN

Risk management during distribution and supply chain operations is crucial for ensuring the safe and effective delivery of medical devices to end-users. This phase involves managing risks associated with transportation, storage, handling, and traceability of devices throughout the supply chain. By implementing appropriate risk management strategies, manufacturers can mitigate potential hazards and ensure the quality and integrity of the devices. Here are key aspects of risk management during distribution and supply chain:

1. **Supplier Management:**

   - **Supplier Qualification:** Implement a robust supplier qualification process to assess the capabilities, reliability, and quality systems of suppliers involved in the distribution and supply chain. This includes evaluating their adherence to regulatory requirements, quality control procedures, and track record.

   - **Supplier Audits:** Conduct periodic audits of suppliers to ensure ongoing compliance with quality and regulatory standards. Assess their handling, storage, and distribution processes to identify potential risks and deviations.

2. **Transportation and Logistics:**

   - **Transportation Risk Assessment:** Perform risk assessments for transportation methods used to distribute medical devices. Consider factors such as temperature control, packaging integrity, security, and handling conditions during transit.

   - **Shipping and Handling Procedures:** Develop and implement standardized shipping and handling procedures to minimize the risk of damage or contamination during transportation. This includes proper packaging, labeling, and instructions to ensure safe and secure delivery.

- **Cold Chain Management:** If applicable, implement appropriate controls for devices requiring temperature-controlled storage and transportation. This includes monitoring temperature conditions, using validated packaging, and ensuring compliance with regulatory requirements.

3. **Storage and Warehousing:**

- **Warehouse Management Systems:** Implement robust warehouse management systems to ensure proper storage, inventory control, and traceability of medical devices. This includes maintaining appropriate storage conditions, implementing FIFO (First In, First Out) practices, and tracking expiration dates.

- **Risk-based Storage Controls:** Identify and mitigate potential risks associated with storage conditions, such as temperature, humidity, light exposure, and handling. Implement risk-based controls, including monitoring and alarms, to maintain the required storage conditions.

4. **Traceability and Serialization:**

- **Unique Device Identification (UDI):** Implement a robust system for assigning and tracking unique device identifiers (UDIs) throughout the supply chain. This enables effective traceability and recall management, allowing for prompt identification and isolation of potentially affected devices.

- **Serialization and Barcoding:** Apply serialization and barcoding techniques to individual device units and packaging to enhance traceability, reduce counterfeiting risks, and facilitate accurate inventory management.

5. **Product Returns and Recalls:**

- **Return and Recall Procedures:** Establish clear procedures for handling product returns and managing recalls. This includes mechanisms for promptly identifying and addressing non-conforming or potentially defective devices, coordinating with relevant stakeholders, and initiating appropriate corrective actions.

- **Communication and Notification:** Maintain effective communication channels with regulatory authorities, distributors, healthcare providers, and end-users to communicate recall notifications promptly, safety alerts, and other relevant information.

6. **Regulatory Compliance:**

- **Compliance Monitoring:** Continuously monitor and ensure compliance with relevant regulatory requirements, including Good Distribution Practices (GDP) and any specific regional or international regulations governing medical device distribution.

- **Regulatory Reporting:** Adhere to reporting requirements for adverse events, product complaints, or other incidents as specified by regulatory authorities. This includes timely reporting of incidents that may impact the safety or performance of distributed devices.

By effectively managing risks during distribution and supply chain operations, medical device manufacturers can ensure the integrity, quality, and safety of their products throughout the entire supply chain. This helps protect patients and end-users from potential hazards, supports regulatory compliance, and maintains trust in the reliability and effectiveness of the devices.

5.4 RISK MANAGEMENT DURING POST-MARKET SURVEILLANCE

Risk management during post-market surveillance is a critical aspect of ensuring the ongoing safety and performance of medical devices after they have been placed on the market. It involves systematic monitoring, analysis, and management of potential risks and safety issues that may arise during the device's lifecycle. By effectively managing risks in the post-market phase, manufacturers can take proactive measures to address safety concerns, make necessary improvements, and maintain compliance with regulatory requirements. Here are key aspects of risk management during post-market surveillance:

1. **Adverse Event Reporting:**

   - **Adverse Event Monitoring:** Establish processes for monitoring and capturing adverse events, including incidents, complaints, and other safety-related information associated using the medical device. This includes proactive surveillance through various channels, such as user feedback, complaint databases, clinical studies, literature reviews, and regulatory databases.

   - **Adverse Event Assessment:** Evaluate reported adverse events to determine the severity, frequency, and potential impact on patient safety and device performance. Classify and prioritize events based on their significance and likelihood of occurrence.

2. **Post-Market Data Analysis:**

   - **Trend Analysis:** Conduct regular analysis of post-market data to identify emerging patterns, trends, or signals that may indicate potential risks or safety issues. Use statistical methods and data mining techniques to identify and investigate potential correlations or associations.

   - **Signal Detection:** Implement signal detection processes to identify and evaluate signals that may indicate previously unknown or unexpected risks associated with the device. This involves systematic analysis of post-market data and the application of statistical and epidemiological methods to detect potential safety signals.

3. **Post-Market Surveillance Studies:**

   - **Post-Market Clinical Follow-up (PMCF):** Conduct PMCF studies to collect additional clinical data and real-world evidence on the device's safety and performance in routine clinical practice. These studies help assess the long-term performance, identify potential risks, and validate the device's safety and effectiveness.

   - **Post-Market Surveillance Plans:** Develop and implement post-market surveillance plans that outline the specific activities and methods for monitoring the device's performance and safety in the post-market phase. These plans should align with regulatory requirements and take into account the device's risk profile, intended use, and target population.

4. **Risk Assessment and Risk Control:**

   - **Risk Re-evaluation:** Periodically re-evaluate the identified risks associated with the device based on the post-market surveillance data, including adverse events, complaints, and other safety-related information. Assess the significance and potential impact of these risks on patient safety and device performance.

   - **Risk Control Measures:** Implement appropriate risk control measures based on the findings of the post-market surveillance. This may include design modifications, labeling updates, post-market studies, training and education programs, or additional warnings and precautions to mitigate identified risks.

5. **Communication and Reporting:**

   - **Regulatory Reporting:** Comply with regulatory reporting requirements for adverse events, field safety corrective actions, and other incidents as specified by the regulatory authorities. Ensure timely and accurate reporting of safety-related information to the relevant regulatory agencies.

   - **Communication with Stakeholders:** Maintain effective communication channels with healthcare professionals, patients, regulatory authorities, and other relevant stakeholders. Provide timely updates on safety-related information, including safety alerts, recalls, and corrective actions. Respond promptly to inquiries and address any safety concerns or questions raised by stakeholders.

6. **Post-Market Quality Management:**

   - **Post-Market Quality Systems:** Maintain robust post-market quality systems to ensure ongoing compliance with quality and regulatory requirements. This includes implementing processes for complaint handling, product tracking, trend analysis, and CAPA (Corrective and Preventive Actions).

- **Post-Market Surveillance Plan Updates:** Periodically review and update the post-market surveillance plan to incorporate new knowledge, changes in the device's risk profile, and emerging regulatory requirements.

By effectively managing risks during post-market surveillance, medical device manufacturers can proactively identify and address safety issues, improve device performance, and ensure the continued safety and effectiveness of their products. This contributes to patient safety, regulatory compliance, and the overall success of the device in the market.

5.5 RISK MANAGEMENT FOR LEGACY DEVICES

Risk management for legacy devices refers to the process of assessing and mitigating risks associated with medical devices that were developed and placed on the market before the implementation of comprehensive risk management standards and regulations. These devices may not have undergone the same level of risk analysis and control measures as newer devices designed in accordance with current standards.

Managing risks for legacy devices is important to ensure their continued safety and effectiveness, especially considering that new information or adverse events may emerge over time. Here are key considerations for risk management of legacy devices:

1. **Risk Assessment:**

   - **Review Existing Data:** Gather and review all available data related to the device, including post-market surveillance data, adverse event reports, clinical studies, and any other relevant information.

   - **Identify Potential Hazards:** Identify and evaluate potential hazards associated with the device. This may include analyzing device design, materials, manufacturing processes, and known safety concerns.

- **Consider Clinical Use:** Assess the device's performance and safety in the context of its clinical use, including patient population, indications, and potential misuse or off-label use.

2. **Risk Control Measures:**

   - **Identify Gaps:** Determine any gaps in the existing risk control measures for the legacy device. Compare the device's current risk profile with the requirements outlined in relevant standards and regulations.

   - **Implement Mitigation Strategies:** Develop and implement risk control measures to address identified gaps. This may involve updating labeling, providing additional warnings or precautions, modifying design or manufacturing processes, or conducting post-market surveillance studies to collect additional safety data.

3. **Post-Market Surveillance:**

   - **Enhance Monitoring:** Establish a robust post-market surveillance plan specifically for legacy devices. This includes monitoring adverse events, complaints, and other safety-related information to identify new risks or safety concerns that may arise over time.

   - **Reporting and Communication:** Ensure compliance with regulatory reporting requirements for legacy devices. Promptly report any safety-related information, recalls, or corrective actions to regulatory authorities and communicate relevant updates to healthcare professionals, patients, and other stakeholders.

4. **Risk-Benefit Analysis:**

   - **Evaluate Risk-Benefit Profile:** Perform a comprehensive risk-benefit analysis to determine if the benefits of the legacy device outweigh the identified risks. Consider factors such as the availability of alternative devices, clinical need, patient population, and the device's performance track record.

   - **Risk Communication:** Clearly communicate the known risks associated with the legacy device to healthcare professionals and patients. Provide updated instructions, warnings, and precautions to ensure safe and appropriate use.

5. **Post-Market Actions:**

   - **Corrective Actions:** Implement appropriate corrective actions based on the identified risks and risk control measures. This may involve design modifications, manufacturing process improvements, labeling updates, or training programs for healthcare professionals.

   - **Legacy Device Retirement:** Evaluate the need for retiring the legacy device from the market if the risks outweigh the benefits or if more advanced and safer alternatives are available. This decision should consider the impact on patients, the healthcare system, and regulatory requirements.

6. **Collaboration and Compliance:**

   - **Collaboration with Regulatory Authorities:** Maintain open communication and collaboration with regulatory authorities regarding risk management activities for legacy devices. Seek guidance and input to ensure compliance with relevant regulations and expectations.

   - **Compliance with Updated Standards:** Strive to align the risk management practices for legacy devices with the latest standards and guidelines to the extent feasible and appropriate.

By applying risk management principles to legacy devices, manufacturers can enhance patient safety, address potential risks, and ensure continued regulatory compliance. It is important to balance the benefits and risks associated with these devices and take appropriate actions to manage risks throughout their remaining life span in the market.

RISK MANAGEMENT FOR UNIQUE DEVICE IDENTIFICATION (UDI) SYSTEM

Risk management for the Unique Device Identification (UDI) system is essential to ensure the accurate identification and traceability of medical devices throughout their lifecycle. The UDI system provides a unique identifier for each medical device, allowing for improved product tracking, recalls, adverse event reporting, and post-market surveillance. Here are key considerations for risk management in relation to the UDI system (Figure 6.1):

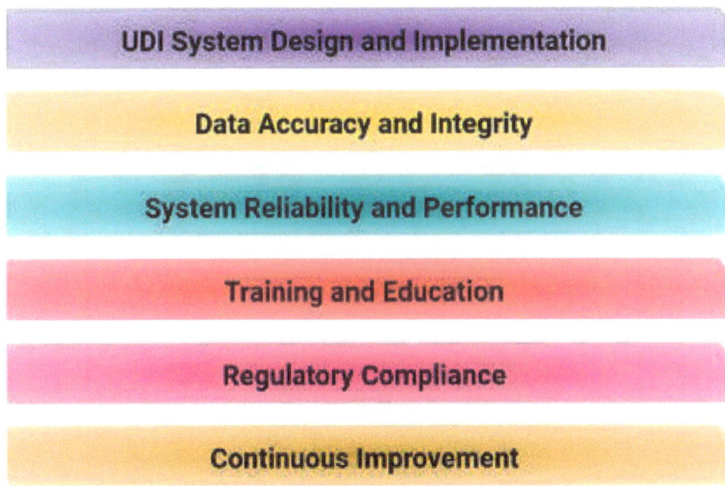

FIGURE 6.1: RISK MANAGEMENT IN RELATION TO THE UDI SYSTEM

1. **UDI System Design and Implementation:**
   - **Risk Identification:** Identify potential risks associated with the design, implementation, and operation of the UDI system. This may include risks related to data accuracy, system interoperability, human errors, and technical failures.
   - **Risk Analysis:** Assess the severity and likelihood of identified risks to prioritize mitigation efforts. Consider the impact of risks on patient safety, data integrity, regulatory compliance, and the effectiveness of the UDI system.

2. **Data Accuracy and Integrity:**
   - **Data Validation:** Implement mechanisms to ensure the accuracy and integrity of UDI data, including data validation checks, verification processes, and error correction procedures.
   - **System Integration:** Ensure seamless integration of the UDI system with other relevant systems, such as electronic health records (EHRs) and inventory management systems. This reduces the risk of data discrepancies and improves the efficiency and accuracy of data exchange.

3. **System Reliability and Performance:**
   - **System Validation:** Conduct thorough testing and validation of the UDI system to ensure its reliability and performance. This includes stress testing, scenario testing, and assessing system response under different operational conditions.
   - **Backup and Recovery:** Implement appropriate backup and recovery mechanisms to safeguard UDI data in the event of system failures, power outages, or other unforeseen circumstances. This minimizes the risk of data loss and ensures the continuity of the UDI system's operation.

4. **Training and Education:**
   - **User Training:** Provide comprehensive training programs for stakeholders involved in the use and management of the UDI system. This includes healthcare professionals, device manufacturers,

regulatory authorities, and system administrators. Training should cover proper UDI data entry, system navigation, and understanding the significance of UDI in patient care and safety.

- **Awareness Programs:** Conduct awareness programs to educate healthcare professionals and end-users about the importance of UDI, its benefits, and how to utilize UDI information for patient safety, product tracking, and adverse event reporting.

5. **Regulatory Compliance:**

- **UDI Regulations:** Ensure compliance with applicable UDI regulations and requirements, such as those outlined by regulatory authorities like the U.S. Food and Drug Administration (FDA) and the European Union Medical Device Regulation (EU MDR). Stay updated with any changes or updates to the UDI regulatory landscape.

- **Audits and Inspections:** Prepare for audits and inspections related to UDI compliance. Maintain proper documentation, record-keeping, and traceability to demonstrate adherence to UDI requirements.

6. **Continuous Improvement:**

- **Monitoring and Feedback:** Implement mechanisms for ongoing monitoring and feedback to identify potential issues or areas for improvement in the UDI system. This may involve gathering user feedback, conducting periodic system audits, and analyzing data quality and usability metrics.

- **Corrective Actions:** Take prompt corrective actions to address identified issues and improve the UDI system. This may involve system updates, process improvements, additional training, or enhancements to data management procedures.

By effectively managing risks associated with the UDI system, medical device manufacturers, healthcare providers, and regulatory authorities can harness the full potential of UDI in improving patient safety, enhancing product traceability, and facilitating effective post-market surveillance. Proper risk management ensures the accurate and reliable identification of medical devices, contributing to better patient outcomes and regulatory compliance.

6.1 INTRODUCTION TO UDI

Unique Device Identification (UDI) is a system implemented in the healthcare industry to provide a unique identifier for medical devices. It is a globally recognized standard that enables the unambiguous identification and traceability of medical devices throughout their lifecycle, from manufacturing to post-market use. The UDI system aims to enhance patient safety, facilitate effective device tracking and recalls, improve post-market surveillance, and support regulatory compliance.

The UDI consists of a unique alphanumeric code that includes both device-specific and production-related information. It is typically encoded in both human-readable and machine-readable formats, such as barcodes or data matrix codes (Figure 6.2). The UDI contains the following key elements:

1. **Device Identifier (DI):** The DI is a fixed portion of the UDI that identifies the specific version or model of the device. It includes information such as the device name, model number, and any variant or configuration details.

2. **Production Identifier (PI):** The PI is a variable portion of the UDI that contains information about the device's production or manufacturing details. It includes details such as the lot or batch number, serial number, manufacturing date, and expiration date.

Figure 6.2: UDI

The UDI serves as a globally unique identifier for each medical device, enabling stakeholders to access important information about the device, such as its specifications, manufacturer details, and regulatory approvals. The UDI system provides several benefits:

1. **Improved Patient Safety:** UDI facilitates accurate identification of medical devices used in patient care, reducing the risk of errors, such as selecting the wrong device or administering the wrong medication. It enhances patient safety by ensuring the right device is used for the right patient at the right time.

2. **Enhanced Device Tracking and Recalls:** UDI enables efficient tracking of medical devices throughout the supply chain, from manufacturing to patient use. In the event of a safety issue or product recall, UDI allows for rapid and precise identification of affected devices, minimizing the impact on patient safety and facilitating timely corrective actions.

3. **Effective Post-Market Surveillance:** UDI enables better monitoring and analysis of device performance and safety in real-world clinical settings. It supports post-market surveillance activities, such as adverse event reporting, signal detection, and trend analysis, leading to improved identification of potential risks and better patient outcomes.

4. **Regulatory Compliance:** UDI is a regulatory requirement in many countries and regions, including the United States (FDA UDI Rule) and the European Union (EU MDR). Compliance with UDI regulations ensures that medical device manufacturers meet the regulatory standards and facilitates market access for their products.

The UDI system is applicable to a wide range of medical devices, including implantable devices, diagnostic equipment, surgical instruments, and consumer healthcare products. It is a powerful tool that enables stakeholders, including healthcare professionals, patients, regulatory authorities, and manufacturers, to access accurate and standardized information about medical devices, promoting patient safety and efficient device management throughout the healthcare system.

6.2 INTEGRATION OF UDI WITH RISK MANAGEMENT

The integration of Unique Device Identification (UDI) with risk management is crucial for effective medical device safety and regulatory compliance. By incorporating UDI data into the risk management process, manufacturers and stakeholders can better identify, evaluate, and mitigate risks associated with medical devices. Here are key aspects of integrating UDI with risk management:

1. **Risk Identification:** UDI can play a significant role in identifying device-related risks. The unique identifier allows for accurate tracking and identification of specific devices, facilitating the collection of data on device performance, adverse events, and safety concerns. UDI data can help identify patterns and trends, enabling early detection of potential risks.

2. **Risk Assessment:** UDI information, particularly the Device Identifier (DI) and Production Identifier (PI), provides valuable data for risk assessment. The DI offers details about the device, including its model, variant, and configuration, which can influence its safety and performance characteristics. The PI, such as the lot or batch number, enables traceability and investigation into specific manufacturing or production-related risks.

3. **Risk Control:** UDI can aid in implementing risk control measures. The UDI system allows for effective tracking of devices throughout the supply chain, enabling targeted interventions or corrective actions if risks are identified. It facilitates efficient device recalls by precisely identifying affected devices and minimizing potential harm to patients.

4. **Post-Market Surveillance:** UDI enhances post-market surveillance activities, which are essential for ongoing risk management. By associating UDI with adverse event reports and post-market surveillance data, manufacturers and regulatory authorities can conduct more accurate signal detection and trend analysis. UDI also enables the monitoring of device performance, safety, and efficacy in real-world clinical settings.

5. **Recall Management:** UDI plays a critical role in managing device recalls. The unique identifier allows for swift and precise identification of affected devices, minimizing the time and effort required to locate and retrieve specific products from the market. UDI data aids in effectively communicating recall information to healthcare professionals, patients, and other stakeholders, ensuring the appropriate actions are taken promptly.

6. **Regulatory Compliance:** UDI is a regulatory requirement in various regions, such as the United States and the European Union. Integrating UDI with risk management ensures compliance with regulatory standards. Risk management processes, including risk assessment, control measures, and post-market surveillance, should consider UDI requirements and align with regulatory expectations.

By integrating UDI with risk management, manufacturers and stakeholders can enhance patient safety, improve device traceability, and streamline regulatory compliance. UDI data provides critical insights into device-related risks, enabling more informed decision-making, targeted risk mitigation strategies, and efficient post-market surveillance. It strengthens the overall risk management process and supports the continuous improvement of medical device safety and performance.

6.3 UDI AND TRACEABILITY FOR RISK MANAGEMENT

Unique Device Identification (UDI) and traceability are closely linked to risk management in the medical device industry. UDI and traceability play a crucial role in identifying, tracking, and managing risks associated with medical devices throughout their lifecycle. Here's how UDI and traceability contribute to risk management:

1. **Device Identification:** UDI provides a unique identifier for each medical device, enabling accurate and unambiguous identification. The UDI includes device-specific information, such as the model, variant, and configuration, which aids in identifying and assessing device-related risks. Proper device identification is essential for effective risk

management as it ensures that risks are attributed to the correct device and not misidentified or overlooked.

2. **Product Traceability:** UDI enables comprehensive product traceability, allowing the tracking of medical devices throughout their entire lifecycle. Traceability encompasses the ability to identify and trace devices from manufacturing to distribution, use, and even post-market activities. By capturing and maintaining UDI-related data at each stage, traceability supports risk management by facilitating the identification of potential risks, monitoring device performance, and enabling timely interventions when necessary.

3. **Risk Assessment and Evaluation:** UDI and traceability data contribute to risk assessment and evaluation processes. By associating UDI with specific device batches, lots, or serial numbers, manufacturers can retrieve relevant data for risk analysis. This includes information on manufacturing processes, materials used, and historical performance data. Traceability data assists in evaluating the severity and likelihood of identified risks, enabling informed decision-making regarding risk mitigation strategies.

4. **Effective Recall Management:** UDI and traceability are instrumental in managing device recalls. In the event of safety issues or product defects, UDI enables swift and precise identification of affected devices. By leveraging traceability data, manufacturers can efficiently locate and retrieve specific devices from the market, minimizing potential harm to patients. UDI and traceability support recall management by facilitating communication, notification, and tracking of recalled devices, ensuring effective risk mitigation.

5. **Post-Market Surveillance:** UDI and traceability enhance post-market surveillance activities, which are critical for ongoing risk management. By capturing UDI-related data in adverse event reporting and post-market surveillance systems, manufacturers and regulatory authorities can identify trends, patterns, and signals of potential risks. This enables proactive risk assessment, evaluation, and implementation of necessary control measures to improve patient safety and device performance.

6. **Regulatory Compliance:** UDI and traceability are regulatory requirements in many regions. Compliance with UDI regulations ensures that medical device manufacturers meet specific standards related to device identification and traceability. Aligning with regulatory requirements supports effective risk management by ensuring that devices are adequately identified, tracked, and monitored throughout their lifecycle.

UDI and traceability provide a systematic approach to risk management in the medical device industry. By incorporating UDI and traceability into risk management processes, stakeholders can enhance patient safety, streamline recall management, facilitate post-market surveillance, and ensure compliance with regulatory requirements. These practices contribute to overall risk mitigation and continuous improvement in the safety and performance of medical devices.

6.4 UDI DATABASE AND RISK MANAGEMENT

The establishment and utilization of a UDI database can significantly contribute to effective risk management in the medical device industry. A UDI database serves as a centralized repository of information related to medical devices and their unique identifiers, providing a valuable resource for risk assessment, evaluation, and mitigation. Here's how a UDI database supports risk management:

1. **Data Consolidation:** A UDI database brings together UDI-related data from various sources, including manufacturers, regulatory authorities, healthcare facilities, and post-market surveillance systems. By consolidating this data into a single database, it enables comprehensive analysis and evaluation of device-related risks. This centralized repository allows for the integration of UDI data with other risk management information, facilitating a holistic approach to risk assessment and decision-making.

2. **Risk Identification and Analysis:** The UDI database provides a wealth of information that can be leveraged for risk identification and analysis.

By associating UDI data with adverse event reports, post-market surveillance data, and other relevant risk-related information, patterns and trends can be identified. This helps in the early detection and assessment of potential risks associated with specific devices, product lines, or manufacturers.

3. **Enhanced Traceability:** A UDI database enhances traceability by capturing and maintaining comprehensive records of device identification, production, distribution, and utilization. This traceability data assists in tracking devices throughout their lifecycle, enabling efficient identification of devices subject to safety concerns or recalls. The UDI database supports traceability-related risk management activities, such as recall management, investigation of manufacturing-related risks, and monitoring of device performance.

4. **Real-Time Monitoring:** A UDI database can be designed to provide real-time monitoring and updates on device-related risks. By integrating with other systems, such as adverse event reporting or post-market surveillance platforms, the database can capture and analyze risk-related data in real-time. This allows for proactive risk management measures, such as timely signal detection, risk evaluation, and implementation of risk control strategies.

5. **Regulatory Compliance:** A UDI database can assist in meeting regulatory requirements related to UDI and risk management. It allows manufacturers to maintain accurate and up-to-date UDI information, ensuring compliance with regulatory standards. The database can also facilitate the exchange of UDI data with regulatory authorities, supporting their risk management and surveillance activities.

6. **Knowledge Base for Decision-Making:** A UDI database serves as a knowledge base for risk management decision-making. It provides a comprehensive source of information on medical devices, including their specifications, manufacturing details, regulatory approvals, and associated risks. This knowledge base supports informed decision-

making regarding risk mitigation strategies, recall management, and overall device safety.

By establishing and utilizing a UDI database, stakeholders in the medical device industry can leverage the power of data to enhance risk management practices. The database enables efficient data consolidation, risk identification, traceability, real-time monitoring, and compliance with regulatory requirements. It serves as a valuable tool for risk assessment, evaluation, and decision-making, ultimately contributing to improved patient safety and the effective management of device-related risks.

CHAPTER 7

RISK MANAGEMENT AND POST-MARKET SURVEILLANCE

Risk management and post-market surveillance are closely interconnected processes in the medical device industry (as shown in Figure 7.1). While risk management focuses on identifying, evaluating, and mitigating risks associated with medical devices throughout their lifecycle, post-market surveillance plays a critical role in monitoring device performance, detecting adverse events, and ensuring ongoing patient safety. Here's how risk management and post-market surveillance are related:

1. **Risk Identification:** Post-market surveillance activities, such as adverse event reporting and complaint handling, contribute to the identification of device-related risks. Real-world data and feedback from healthcare professionals, patients, and other stakeholders help in recognizing potential safety issues, malfunctions, or performance concerns. These identified risks feed into the risk management process, where they are further assessed and analyzed.

2. **Risk Evaluation:** Post-market surveillance data provides valuable insights for risk evaluation. By analyzing adverse event reports, complaint data, and other post-market information, manufacturers can assess the severity, frequency, and potential consequences of identified risks. This evaluation helps in determining the level of risk associated with specific devices and informs risk management decision-making.

3. **Risk Control:** Post-market surveillance plays a crucial role in implementing risk control measures. If device-related risks are identified through surveillance activities, appropriate actions can be taken to mitigate those risks. This may include implementing corrective actions, issuing safety communications, modifying device labeling or instructions for use, or even initiating device recalls. The goal is to control effectively and manage risks to ensure patient safety.

4. **Signal Detection and Trend Analysis:** Post-market surveillance data aids in signal detection and trend analysis, which are vital for proactive risk management. By systematically analyzing reported adverse events, complaint trends, and other post-market data, manufacturers can identify potential emerging risks or patterns that may require further investigation. This helps in staying ahead of potential safety concerns and taking necessary risk mitigation measures.

5. **Post-Market Surveillance as a Feedback Loop:** Post-market surveillance acts as a feedback loop for risk management. The data collected during surveillance activities provides valuable feedback on the effectiveness of risk control measures implemented during the pre-market phase. It helps in assessing the performance of medical devices in real-world settings and informs continuous improvement efforts, including design changes, manufacturing process improvements, and risk mitigation strategies.

6. **Regulatory Compliance:** Post-market surveillance is often a regulatory requirement to ensure ongoing compliance with safety and performance standards. Regulatory authorities expect manufacturers to have robust post-market surveillance systems in place to monitor device safety and effectiveness. Compliance with post-market surveillance requirements supports overall risk management efforts and facilitates adherence to regulatory obligations.

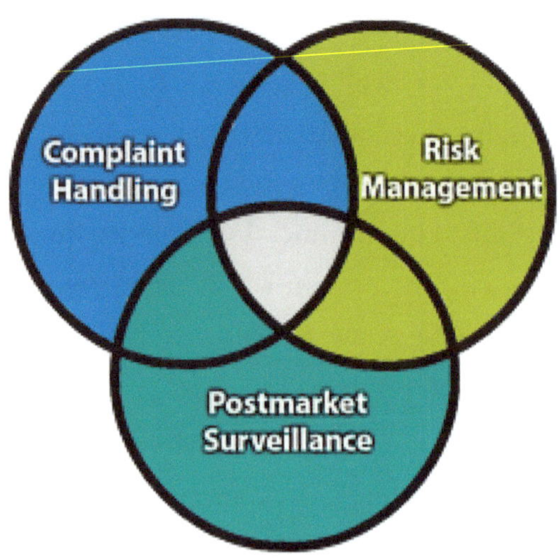

FIGURE 7.1: INTEGRATION OF RISK MANAGEMENT WITH POST-MARKET SURVEILLANCE

By integrating risk management with post-market surveillance, manufacturers can proactively identify, evaluate, and control risks associated with medical devices in the real-world setting. The continuous monitoring of device performance and the timely detection of safety concerns through post-market surveillance help in implementing effective risk mitigation measures, enhancing patient safety, and ensuring regulatory compliance. It is a cyclical process that feeds back into risk management, driving continuous improvement and the safe use of medical devices.

7.1 IMPORTANCE OF POST-MARKET SURVEILLANCE

Post-market surveillance is of paramount importance in the medical device industry. It plays a crucial role in ensuring patient safety, monitoring device performance, and facilitating continuous improvement. Here are some key reasons why post-market surveillance is important:

1. **Patient Safety:** Post-market surveillance is essential for monitoring the safety of medical devices once they are in use by patients. It helps identify adverse events, malfunctions, or any other issues that may

pose a risk to patients' health and well-being. By promptly detecting and addressing potential safety concerns, post-market surveillance contributes to enhancing patient safety.

2. **Real-World Performance Monitoring:** Post-market surveillance provides an opportunity to evaluate the performance of medical devices in real-world settings. It allows manufacturers to gather data on how devices are being used, their effectiveness, and any challenges encountered by users. This data helps in assessing the device's performance in diverse patient populations and clinical environments, supporting evidence-based decision-making and product improvements.

3. **Early Detection of Safety Signals:** Post-market surveillance enables the early detection of safety signals, including emerging risks or patterns of adverse events. By systematically collecting and analyzing data from multiple sources such as adverse event reports, complaint data, and registries, manufacturers can identify potential safety issues that were not evident during pre-market testing. Early detection allows for timely risk assessment and implementation of appropriate measures to mitigate risks.

4. **Regulatory Compliance:** Regulatory authorities require manufacturers to have robust post-market surveillance systems in place as a condition for marketing approval and ongoing compliance. Compliance with post-market surveillance regulations ensures that manufacturers meet their obligations to monitor the safety and performance of their devices. Non-compliance can lead to regulatory penalties, loss of market authorization, or reputational damage.

5. **Continuous Improvement:** Post-market surveillance provides valuable feedback for continuous improvement efforts. By analyzing post-market data, manufacturers can identify areas for device enhancements, design modifications, or process improvements. This feedback loop helps in addressing device-related issues, optimizing performance, and enhancing the overall quality of medical devices.

6. **Risk Mitigation and Recall Management:** Post-market surveillance is vital for effective risk mitigation and recall management. It enables the identification of safety concerns or defects that may require corrective actions or device recalls. By monitoring adverse events, complaints, and other post-market data, manufacturers can take prompt action to mitigate risks and protect patients from potential harm.

7. **Regulatory Reporting and Transparency:** Post-market surveillance data is often used for regulatory reporting purposes, including submission of periodic safety reports and post-market surveillance updates. It contributes to regulatory transparency by providing regulators, healthcare professionals, and the public with important information on device safety and performance. This transparency builds trust and confidence in the medical device industry.

Overall, post-market surveillance is critical for ensuring the ongoing safety and effectiveness of medical devices. It helps in identifying and mitigating risks, monitoring device performance, and driving continuous improvement. By actively engaging in post-market surveillance activities, manufacturers can enhance patient safety, comply with regulatory requirements, and contribute to the overall advancement of the medical device industry.

7.2 POST-MARKET SURVEILLANCE PROCESSES

Post-market surveillance processes are essential for monitoring the safety and performance of medical devices once they are on the market. These processes involve the systematic collection, analysis, and evaluation of data related to adverse events, complaints, and other post-market information. Here are the key steps involved in post-market surveillance (as mentioned in Table 7.1 and Figure 7.2):

TABLE 7.1: POST-MARKET SURVEILLANCE PROCESSES

Post-Market Surveillance Processes
1. Data Collection
2. Data Analysis
3. Risk Assessment
4. Risk Mitigation
5. Trend Analysis and Signal Detection
6. Reporting and Documentation
7. Continuous Improvement

This table summarizes the main steps involved in post-market surveillance. Each process contributes to the overall goal of monitoring device safety, identifying risks, and ensuring ongoing product quality.

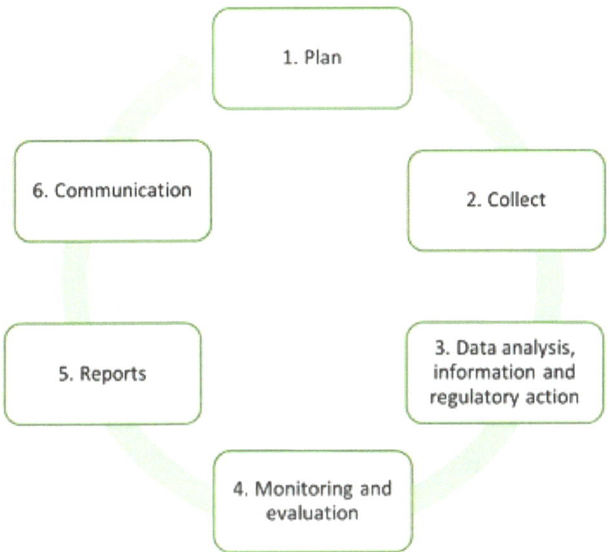

FIGURE 7.2: POST-MARKET SURVEILLANCE PROCESSES

1. **Data Collection:** The first step in post-market surveillance is the collection of relevant data. This includes adverse event reports, complaints from healthcare professionals and patients, product performance data, and any other post-market information sources.

Data can be obtained from various channels such as voluntary reporting systems, user feedback, registries, and clinical studies.

2. **Data Analysis:** Once the data is collected, it needs to be analyzed to identify any potential safety concerns or trends. This involves reviewing and categorizing the data based on factors such as the type of adverse event, severity, frequency, and associated patient population. Data analysis techniques such as statistical analysis, data mining, and signal detection methods may be employed to identify patterns or signals that warrant further investigation.

3. **Risk Assessment:**

    The next step is to assess the identified risks based on the collected data. This involves evaluating the severity and likelihood of harm associated with the risks. Risk assessment methods such as risk matrices, risk scoring systems, or qualitative assessments may be used to determine the level of risk posed by the device. This assessment helps prioritize risks for further action.

4. **Risk Mitigation:** If risks are identified through the assessment process, appropriate risk mitigation measures should be implemented. This may include issuing safety communications, updating device labeling or instructions for use, implementing corrective actions, or initiating a device recall. The aim is to minimize or eliminate the identified risks and ensure patient safety.

5. **Trend Analysis and Signal Detection:** Post-market surveillance involves ongoing trend analysis and signal detection to identify any emerging risks or safety signals. This entails monitoring the collected data over time to detect any new patterns, changes in adverse event rates, or unexpected device performance issues. Regular data review and analysis enable the timely identification and proactive management of potential risks.

6. **Reporting and Documentation:** Post-market surveillance activities require comprehensive reporting and documentation. This includes preparing periodic safety reports, post-market surveillance updates, and

other regulatory submissions as required by the applicable regulatory authorities. Accurate and timely reporting ensures compliance with regulatory obligations and facilitates transparency in communicating device safety information.

7. **Continuous Improvement:** Post-market surveillance serves as a feedback loop for continuous improvement efforts. It provides valuable insights into device performance and safety, which can inform product enhancements, design modifications, and manufacturing process improvements. Manufacturers can use the information obtained through post-market surveillance to drive continuous improvement and ensure the ongoing quality and safety of their devices.

By following these post-market surveillance processes, manufacturers can effectively monitor the performance and safety of medical devices in real-world settings, detect and mitigate risks, and contribute to patient safety and overall product improvement.

7.3 FEEDBACK LOOPS FOR CONTINUOUS RISK MANAGEMENT

Feedback loops play a crucial role in continuous risk management within the medical device industry. These loops enable the collection of valuable information, analysis of data, and implementation of necessary actions to mitigate risks throughout the lifecycle of a medical device. Here's an overview of the feedback loops involved in continuous risk management:

1. **Post-Market Surveillance Feedback Loop:** (as summarized in Table 7.2)

   - **Data Collection:** Post-market surveillance activities gather data on adverse events, complaints, user feedback, and other post-market information.

   - **Data Analysis:** Collected data is analyzed to identify potential safety concerns, patterns, or emerging risks.

   - **Risk Assessment:** The identified risks are assessed based on severity, likelihood, and impact on patient safety.

- **Risk Mitigation:** Appropriate actions, such as safety communications, labeling updates, or recalls, are implemented to mitigate identified risks.

- **Continuous Improvement:** Lessons learned from post-market surveillance inform product enhancements, design modifications, and risk control strategies.

TABLE 7.2: POST-MARKET SURVEILLANCE FEEDBACK LOOP

Stage	Activities
Data Collection	- Collect adverse events, complaints, and feedback
	- Obtain post-market information sources
Data Analysis	- Analyze collected data for safety concerns
	- Identify patterns or emerging risks
Risk Assessment	- Evaluate risks based on severity and likelihood
	- Assess impact on patient safety
Risk Mitigation	- Implement safety communications
	- Update labeling or initiate recalls
Continuous Improvement	- Incorporate findings into product enhancements
	- Modify design or risk control strategies

2. **Feedback Loop from Clinical Trials and Studies:** (as summarized in Table 7.3)

   - **Data Collection:** Clinical trials and studies generate data on device performance, safety, and effectiveness in controlled settings.

   - **Data Analysis:** Analyzing clinical trial data helps identify potential risks, device-related issues, or adverse events.

   - **Risk Assessment:** The risks identified during clinical trials are evaluated and incorporated into the risk management process.

- **Risk Mitigation:** Risk control measures are implemented based on the findings from clinical trials to enhance device safety and efficacy.

- **Continuous Improvement:** Feedback from clinical trials informs ongoing product development and risk management strategies.

TABLE 7.3: FEEDBACK LOOP FROM CLINICAL TRIALS AND STUDIES

Stage	Activities
Data Collection	- Gather data from clinical trials and studies
	- Collect information on device performance
	- Obtain safety and efficacy data
Data Analysis	- Analyze clinical trial data for risks and issues
	- Identify adverse events and safety concerns
Risk Assessment	- Evaluate risks identified during trials
	- Assess impact on patient safety
Risk Mitigation	- Implement risk control measures based on findings
	- Enhance device safety and efficacy
Continuous Improvement	- Incorporate feedback into product development
	- Improve risk management strategies

3. **Manufacturing and Production Feedback Loop:**

- **Data Collection:** Data is collected during manufacturing and production processes, including quality control checks, inspections, and testing.

- **Data Analysis:** Analyzing manufacturing data helps identify any deviations, defects, or quality issues that may impact device safety.

- **Risk Assessment:** The risks associated with manufacturing processes are assessed to determine their potential impact on device safety and performance.

- **Risk Mitigation:** Corrective and preventive actions are implemented to address identified risks and improve manufacturing processes.

- **Continuous Improvement:** Feedback from manufacturing processes informs process optimization and risk control measures.

4. **User Feedback and Complaints Feedback Loop:**

- **Data Collection:** User feedback and complaints provide insights into device performance, user experiences, and potential risks.

- **Data Analysis:** Analyzing user feedback and complaints helps identify common issues, recurring problems, or safety concerns.

- **Risk Assessment:** The risks associated with user feedback and complaints are assessed to determine their impact on device safety.

- **Risk Mitigation:** Corrective actions, user education, or device modifications are implemented based on the findings from user feedback and complaints.

- **Continuous Improvement:** User feedback and complaints drive product improvements, usability enhancements, and risk management strategies.

These feedback loops enable a continuous cycle of information gathering, analysis, risk assessment, risk mitigation, and continuous improvement. By incorporating feedback from various sources, manufacturers can proactively identify and address risks, enhance device safety, and ensure ongoing compliance with regulatory requirements.

7.4 POST-MARKET RISK ANALYSIS AND DECISION MAKING

Post-market risk analysis and decision-making are crucial components of the risk management process in the medical device industry. They involve assessing and evaluating risks associated with devices already on the market, and making informed decisions to mitigate those risks. Here are the key steps involved:

1. **Data Collection:** Gather relevant data from various sources, such as post-market surveillance reports, adverse event databases, user feedback, complaints, and clinical studies.

2. **Data Analysis:** Analyze the collected data to identify patterns, trends, and potential risks associated with the device. This analysis may involve statistical methods, trend analysis, signal detection techniques, and other analytical tools.

3. **Risk Identification:** Identify and document the specific risks associated with the device. This may include known risks, emerging risks, and risks identified through data analysis.

4. **Risk Assessment:** Evaluate the identified risks based on their severity, likelihood, and potential impact on patient safety and device performance. This step helps prioritize risks and determine their significance.

5. **Risk Evaluation:** Assess the identified risks in relation to the risk acceptance criteria established for the device. This involves considering factors such as the intended use, patient population, and overall benefit-risk balance.

6. **Decision-Making:** Based on the risk assessment and evaluation, make informed decisions regarding risk mitigation measures. This may include taking actions such as labeling updates, additional safety precautions, device modifications, or initiating recalls.

7. **Risk Control:** Implement the selected risk mitigation measures to reduce or eliminate the identified risks. This may involve updating instructions for use, implementing new labeling, enhancing training and education, or conducting further studies or tests.

8. **Documentation:** Document all the steps taken, including the risk analysis, evaluation, decision-making, and implemented risk control measures. Maintain thorough records to demonstrate compliance with regulatory requirements and ensure traceability.

9. **Communication:** Communicate the findings, decisions, and actions to relevant stakeholders, including regulatory authorities, healthcare professionals, and users. Timely and effective communication is essential for transparency and ensuring the safety of patients.

10. **Monitoring and Review:** Continuously monitor the effectiveness of the implemented risk control measures and review the post-market performance of the device. This helps identify any new risks or changes in the risk profile and enables iterative improvements in risk management processes.

Post-market risk analysis and decision-making are iterative processes that require ongoing vigilance and continuous improvement. They contribute to the overall goal of ensuring the safety and effectiveness of medical devices throughout their lifecycle in the market.

7.5 POST-MARKET RISK MANAGEMENT REPORTING

Post-market risk management reporting is a critical aspect of the risk management process in the medical device industry. It involves the systematic documentation and communication of post-market risk-related information to relevant stakeholders. Here are the key considerations for post-market risk management reporting:

1. **Reporting Requirements:** Understand the reporting requirements set forth by regulatory authorities and other relevant stakeholders. These requirements may include specific timelines, formats, and content for risk-related reporting.

2. **Report Content:** Include comprehensive information in the risk management reports. This typically involves providing an overview of the device, summarizing post-market surveillance data, describing identified risks and their assessment, outlining risk mitigation measures implemented, and documenting the outcomes and effectiveness of those measures.

3. **Adverse Events Reporting:** Include information on adverse events, complaints, and other incidents related to the device. Report details

such as the nature of the event, its severity, and any actions taken or planned to address it.

4. **Trend Analysis:** Conduct trend analysis to identify patterns, recurring issues, or emerging risks. Report on any notable trends observed and their potential implications on device safety and performance.

5. **Risk Assessment:** Document the risk assessment process and its outcomes. Provide a clear overview of the identified risks, their severity, likelihood, and potential impact on patient safety.

6. **Risk Mitigation Measures:** Report on the risk control measures implemented to mitigate identified risks. Describe the actions taken, such as labeling updates, safety communications, device modifications, or recalls, and provide supporting rationale for these decisions.

7. **Effectiveness Evaluation:** Assess and report on the effectiveness of the implemented risk control measures. Describe any changes in device safety, performance, or user experience resulting from the implemented measures.

8. **Continuous Improvement:** Highlight any lessons learned and continuous improvement initiatives based on post-market surveillance data and risk management findings. Report on any enhancements made to the device design, manufacturing processes, or risk management strategies.

9. **Regulatory Reporting:** Comply with regulatory reporting obligations by submitting required reports to regulatory authorities within the specified timelines. This may include adverse event reporting, periodic safety update reports, or other post-market surveillance reporting requirements.

10. **Stakeholder Communication:** Share the risk management reports with relevant stakeholders, such as regulatory authorities, notified bodies, healthcare professionals, and users. Ensure effective communication to promote transparency and enhance patient safety.

Post-market risk management reporting serves as a mechanism for monitoring device performance, identifying emerging risks, and facilitating ongoing improvements in device safety. By systematically documenting and communicating risk-related information, manufacturers can demonstrate compliance with regulatory requirements, ensure transparency, and contribute to the continuous improvement of their devices.

CHAPTER 8

RISK MANAGEMENT IN A GLOBAL CONTEXT

Risk management in the medical device industry must be conducted in a global context due to the international nature of the industry and the need to comply with various regulatory frameworks. Here are some key considerations for risk management in a global context:

1. **Global Regulatory Frameworks:** Familiarize yourself with the regulatory requirements of different countries and regions where your medical device will be marketed. Understand the specific risk management standards, guidelines, and documentation requirements applicable in each jurisdiction.

2. **Harmonization of Standards:** Recognize the efforts made by regulatory authorities and standardization bodies to harmonize risk management standards and practices. For example, the International Organization for Standardization (ISO) develops globally recognized standards such as ISO 14971, which provide a framework for risk management.

3. **Regional Regulations:** Be aware of regional regulations, such as the European Union's Medical Device Regulation (MDR) and In Vitro Diagnostic Regulation (IVDR), which impose specific risk management obligations. Understand the risk classification criteria and requirements for clinical evaluation, post-market surveillance, and vigilance reporting.

4. **Cultural Factors:** Consider cultural differences when assessing risks and implementing risk mitigation strategies. Patient preferences, healthcare practices, and regulatory attitudes towards risk may vary across different regions and countries. Adapt your risk management approach to align with the cultural context.

5. **Language and Documentation:** Ensure that risk management documentation, such as risk management plans, hazard analyses, and risk management reports, are available in the relevant languages of the target markets. This facilitates effective communication and understanding among stakeholders.

6. **Post-Market Surveillance:** Establish mechanisms for post-market surveillance and adverse event reporting that comply with the requirements of different regulatory authorities. Monitor and analyze post-market data from various regions to identify trends, potential risks, and the need for risk mitigation measures.

7. **International Collaboration:** Engage in international collaborations and partnerships to stay updated on global trends in risk management, share best practices, and learn from experiences in different markets. Participate in industry associations, conferences, and regulatory forums to enhance knowledge sharing and cooperation.

8. **Unique Device Identification (UDI):** Implement a globally recognized UDI system to ensure traceability and facilitate post-market surveillance. UDI allows for easier identification of devices, monitoring of their performance, and effective management of recalls or safety alerts across different markets.

9. **Supply Chain Management:** Evaluate and manage risks associated with the global supply chain, including sourcing of components, manufacturing processes, and distribution networks. Collaborate with suppliers and contract manufacturers to ensure adherence to risk management practices.

10. **Ongoing Compliance Monitoring:** Continuously monitor changes in global regulations, standards, and guidelines to ensure ongoing compliance with evolving requirements. Stay informed about regulatory updates, market surveillance activities, and safety alerts from different jurisdictions.

Managing risks in a global context requires a comprehensive understanding of regulatory landscapes, cultural factors, and market-specific requirements. By incorporating these considerations into risk management processes, medical device manufacturers can navigate global markets effectively, ensure compliance, and prioritize patient safety on a global scale.

8.1 INTERNATIONAL HARMONIZATION OF RISK MANAGEMENT STANDARDS

International harmonization of risk management standards is an important aspect of the medical device industry. It involves aligning risk management practices, methodologies, and requirements across different countries and regions to promote consistency, facilitate trade, and enhance patient safety (discussed in Table 8.1 and 8.2). Here are some key examples of international harmonization efforts in risk management:

1. **International Organization for Standardization (ISO):** The ISO plays a significant role in developing globally recognized risk management standards for the medical device industry. ISO 14971:2019, "Medical devices - Application of risk management to medical devices," provides a comprehensive framework for risk management throughout the entire lifecycle of medical devices.

2. **International Medical Device Regulators Forum (IMDRF):** The IMDRF is a global forum composed of regulatory authorities and industry representatives working towards harmonizing medical device regulations and promoting convergence. The IMDRF has developed guidelines, such as the "Principles of Medical Device Post-Market Surveillance" and the "Essential Principles of Safety and Performance of Medical Devices," which include risk management considerations.

3. **European Union (EU) Regulations:** The EU has made efforts to harmonize risk management practices through regulations such as the Medical Device Regulation (MDR) and the In Vitro Diagnostic Regulation (IVDR). These regulations establish common requirements for risk assessment, risk management, post-market surveillance, and clinical evaluation of medical devices.

4. **Global Harmonization Task Force (GHTF):** The GHTF, now succeeded by the International Medical Device Regulators Forum (IMDRF), aimed to promote international harmonization of medical device regulations. It developed guidance documents, such as the "Essential Principles of Safety and Performance of Medical Devices," which emphasize risk management as a fundamental aspect of device safety.

**TABLE 8.1: GLOBAL HARMONIZATION OF
RISK MANAGEMENT STANDARDS**

Standard/Initiative	Description
ISO 14971:2019	International standard developed by the International Organization for Standardization (ISO) that provides a framework for risk management for medical devices
International Medical Device Regulators Forum (IMDRF)	Global forum comprising regulatory authorities and industry representatives working towards harmonization of medical device regulations
Essential Principles of Safety and Performance of Medical Devices	Guidance documents developed by the Global Harmonization Task Force (GHTF) and the IMDRF, emphasizing risk management as a fundamental aspect of device safety
Harmonized Risk Assessment Templates	Collaborative efforts to develop harmonized risk assessment templates to streamline risk assessment processes across different jurisdictions
Common Terminology	Efforts to establish common terminology and definitions related to risk management, ensuring consistent understanding and communication across borders

5. **Regional Harmonization Efforts:** Various regional bodies and organizations, such as the Association of Southeast Asian Nations (ASEAN) and the Pan American Health Organization (PAHO), have made efforts to harmonize medical device regulations and promote risk management best practices within their respective regions.

TABLE 8.2: REGIONAL HARMONIZATION EFFORTS IN RISK MANAGEMENT

Region/Initiative	Description
European Union (EU)	Regulations such as the Medical Device Regulation (MDR) and the In Vitro Diagnostic Regulation (IVDR) aim to harmonize risk management requirements across EU member states
Association of Southeast Asian Nations (ASEAN)	Collaborative efforts among ASEAN member states to harmonize medical device regulations, including risk management practices
Pan American Health Organization (PAHO)	Harmonization initiatives by PAHO member countries to align medical device regulations and promote best practices in risk management
Mercosur	Regional harmonization efforts among Mercosur member countries in South America, including the harmonization of risk management requirements
Gulf Cooperation Council (GCC)	Harmonization of medical device regulations, including risk management, among GCC member states in the Arabian Peninsula

The goal of international harmonization is to streamline regulatory processes, reduce barriers to trade, and enhance patient safety by promoting consistent and effective risk management practices across different jurisdictions. Harmonized standards and guidelines provide a common language and framework for manufacturers, regulators, and other stakeholders involved in the medical device industry. By adhering to internationally recognized risk management standards, manufacturers can demonstrate compliance, improve product quality, and ensure the safety and effectiveness of their medical devices on a global scale.

8.2 RISK MANAGEMENT CHALLENGES IN GLOBAL MARKETS

Expanding into global markets presents unique challenges for risk management in the medical device industry. Here are some key challenges faced:

1. **Diverse Regulatory Requirements:** Different countries and regions have varying regulatory frameworks and requirements for risk management. Manufacturers must navigate and comply with multiple sets of regulations, which can be complex and time-consuming.

2. **Language and Cultural Differences:** Operating in global markets requires effective communication and understanding of cultural nuances. Language barriers and cultural differences can impact the interpretation and implementation of risk management practices, leading to potential inconsistencies or misunderstandings.

3. **Harmonization and Standardization:** While there are efforts to harmonize risk management standards globally, achieving complete harmonization is challenging. Differences in regulatory expectations, documentation requirements, and risk assessment methodologies may exist, making it difficult for manufacturers to achieve consistent risk management practices across different markets.

4. **Localized Risk Factors:** Each market may have unique risk factors associated with healthcare practices, patient populations, and environmental conditions. Manufacturers must consider and address

these localized risks to ensure the safety and effectiveness of their devices in different regions.

5. **Supply Chain Complexity:** Global supply chains involve various stakeholders, including suppliers, manufacturers, distributors, and service providers. Ensuring effective risk management throughout the supply chain, including risk assessment, control, and communication, can be challenging due to the geographical distribution and diverse regulatory environments.

6. **Post-Market Surveillance:** Monitoring and addressing post-market risks and safety issues become more complex in global markets. Different reporting requirements, varying levels of vigilance systems, and diverse post-market surveillance practices across jurisdictions can pose challenges in capturing and managing post-market safety data.

7. **Training and Education:** Implementing consistent risk management practices across global teams requires comprehensive training and education programs. Ensuring that all personnel involved in risk management processes understand the applicable regulations, standards, and best practices can be a challenge, especially when language and cultural differences are involved.

8. **Legal and Liability Considerations:** Legal and liability frameworks differ across jurisdictions, impacting how manufacturers address and manage risks. Understanding the legal requirements, product liability laws, and potential litigation risks in different markets is crucial for effective risk management.

Addressing these challenges requires a proactive and comprehensive approach to risk management. Manufacturers should stay informed about global regulatory requirements, engage in continuous training and education, establish effective communication channels, and adapt their risk management processes to the specific needs and requirements of each market. Collaboration with local regulatory bodies, consultants, and industry associations can also help navigate the complexities of global risk management.

8.3 LOCALIZATION OF RISK MANAGEMENT PROCESSES

Localization of risk management processes refers to the adaptation and customization of risk management practices to meet the specific requirements and regulations of different countries or regions. It involves tailoring risk management strategies, documentation, and approaches to address local laws, cultural factors, healthcare practices, and patient population characteristics. Here are some key considerations for localizing risk management processes:

1. **Regulatory Compliance:** Each country or region has its own regulatory framework and requirements for risk management in the medical device industry. Manufacturers must understand and comply with the specific regulations governing risk management in each market.

2. **Cultural Factors:** Cultural differences can influence the perception of risk, attitudes towards safety, and communication styles. It is essential to consider cultural nuances when developing risk management strategies and communicating risk-related information to stakeholders.

3. **Language Localization:** Translating risk management documents, labeling, and instructions for use into the local language(s) ensures that users can understand and follow the necessary risk mitigation measures. Localization also includes adapting terminology and ensuring clear and accurate communication.

4. **Local Risk Assessment:** Localizing risk management involves conducting risk assessments that consider local healthcare practices, patient demographics, and environmental factors. Understanding and addressing region-specific risks helps ensure the safety and effectiveness of medical devices in different markets.

5. **Local Regulatory Reporting Requirements:** Adapting risk management processes to comply with local regulatory reporting requirements is crucial. This includes capturing and reporting adverse events, conducting trend analysis, and maintaining vigilance systems specific to each market.

6. **Training and Education:** Providing localized training and education programs to stakeholders, including healthcare professionals, distributors, and end-users, is essential for effective risk management. Localized training materials and programs ensure that individuals understand the specific risks associated with the device and the appropriate risk mitigation measures.

7. **Local Collaboration:** Engaging with local regulatory authorities, industry associations, and healthcare providers helps gain insights into market-specific risks and regulatory expectations. Collaborating with local experts can contribute to a more effective and context-specific approach to risk management.

By localizing risk management processes, medical device manufacturers can address the unique challenges and requirements of different markets, enhance patient safety, and ensure compliance with local regulations. It facilitates effective risk assessment, control, communication, and post-market surveillance, taking into account regional variations and cultural factors.

8.4 RISK MANAGEMENT FOR GLOBAL SUPPLY CHAINS

Managing risk in global supply chains is crucial for the medical device industry to ensure the safety, quality, and timely delivery of products. Here are key considerations for risk management in global supply chains:

1. **Supplier Selection and Qualification:** Thoroughly vetting and selecting suppliers based on their compliance with quality standards, regulatory requirements, and risk management practices. Qualification processes should include supplier audits, assessment of their quality systems, and evaluation of their risk management capabilities.

2. **Supply Chain Visibility:** Establishing robust systems and processes to track and monitor the movement of products throughout the supply chain. This includes implementing technologies like bar coding, RFID, or other traceability systems to ensure visibility and traceability of products at each stage.

3. **Risk Assessment and Management:** Conducting risk assessments at each stage of the supply chain to identify and mitigate potential risks. This includes evaluating risks related to quality, logistics, transportation, storage, and regulatory compliance. Risk mitigation strategies should be implemented to address identified risks effectively.

4. **Supplier Relationship Management:** Building strong relationships with suppliers through effective communication, collaboration, and regular performance evaluations. Clearly defining expectations, sharing risk management practices, and fostering transparency are key to managing risks in supplier relationships.

5. **Contingency Planning:** Developing contingency plans to address potential disruptions in the supply chain, such as natural disasters, transportation issues, or supplier failures. Identifying alternative suppliers, establishing backup inventory, and implementing business continuity plans help minimize the impact of disruptions on the supply chain.

6. **Regulatory Compliance:** Ensuring compliance with regulatory requirements across different regions. Understanding and adhering to local regulations regarding product quality, safety, labeling, and documentation is crucial for managing risks in global supply chains.

7. **Communication and Collaboration:** Establishing effective communication channels with suppliers, logistics partners, and other stakeholders in the supply chain. Regular communication, sharing of information, and collaboration on risk management strategies contribute to improved supply chain resilience.

8. **Continuous Improvement:** Implementing a system of continuous improvement in supply chain risk management. Regularly reviewing and updating risk management strategies, conducting risk assessments, and incorporating lessons learned from incidents or near-misses help enhance the effectiveness of risk management practices.

By adopting a proactive and comprehensive approach to risk management in global supply chains, medical device manufacturers can minimize disruptions, ensure product quality and safety, and maintain compliance with regulatory requirements throughout the supply chain.

8.5 INTERNATIONAL COLLABORATION AND RISK MANAGEMENT

International collaboration plays a vital role in risk management for the medical device industry. Collaborating with global stakeholders, regulatory bodies, and industry associations helps enhance risk management practices and address challenges in a coordinated and harmonized manner. Here are key aspects of international collaboration in risk management:

1. **Harmonization of Standards:** Collaborating with international regulatory bodies, such as the International Organization for Standardization (ISO) and the International Medical Device Regulators Forum (IMDRF), to develop and harmonize risk management standards. Harmonized standards facilitate a consistent approach to risk management globally, reducing complexity for manufacturers operating in multiple markets.

2. **Information Sharing and Best Practices:** Engaging in knowledge sharing and exchanging best practices with global stakeholders. This includes sharing information on risk assessment methodologies, risk control strategies, and post-market surveillance practices. Collaborative platforms, conferences, and industry forums facilitate the exchange of ideas and experiences.

3. **Regulatory Convergence:** Collaborating with regulatory authorities from different countries to align regulations and requirements. Regulatory convergence efforts aim to reduce duplicative efforts, streamline regulatory processes, and harmonize expectations for risk management across jurisdictions. This helps manufacturers navigate global markets more efficiently.

4. **Industry Associations and Networks:** Participating in industry associations and networks that promote collaboration and cooperation among medical device manufacturers, suppliers, and regulatory bodies.

These associations provide platforms for discussions, sharing of experiences, and collaborative initiatives to enhance risk management practices.

5. **Post-Market Surveillance and Vigilance:** Collaborating with regulatory authorities and healthcare providers to improve post-market surveillance and vigilance systems. Sharing adverse event data, conducting trend analysis, and collaborating on signal detection and risk assessment contribute to early detection of safety issues and timely risk mitigation.

6. **Emerging Market Collaboration:** Collaborating with stakeholders in emerging markets to address unique challenges and risks specific to those markets. This includes understanding local healthcare practices, cultural factors, and regulatory requirements. Collaboration can help manufacturers tailor their risk management strategies and products to meet the needs of these markets effectively.

7. **Global Risk Communication:** Collaborating on global risk communication strategies to ensure consistent and accurate information dissemination to healthcare professionals, patients, and other stakeholders. Aligning risk communication practices helps maintain transparency, facilitate understanding, and promote patient safety worldwide.

International collaboration in risk management fosters a global perspective, enables the exchange of knowledge and best practices, and contributes to the development of robust risk management strategies. It helps manufacturers navigate complex regulatory landscapes, mitigate risks effectively, and ensure the safety and quality of medical devices in global markets.

CHAPTER 9

RISK MANAGEMENT AND QUALITY MANAGEMENT SYSTEM

Risk management and quality management systems (QMS) are closely intertwined in the medical device industry. An effective QMS integrates risk management principles and practices to ensure the delivery of safe and high-quality medical devices. Here's how risk management and QMS are interconnected (as discussed in Table 9.1):

1. **Risk-Based Approach:** Both risk management and QMS advocate for a risk-based approach to decision-making. The identification, analysis, and mitigation of risks are central to both disciplines. QMS standards, such as ISO 13485, emphasize the importance of applying risk management throughout the product lifecycle.

2. **Risk Assessment in Design Control:** Risk assessment plays a crucial role in design control, an essential component of QMS. During the design and development of medical devices, risk assessment helps identify potential hazards, evaluate their severity and likelihood, and implement appropriate risk controls to mitigate risks.

3. **Risk-Based Supplier Management:** QMS includes supplier management processes to ensure the quality and reliability of components and materials used in medical devices. Applying risk-based supplier selection, qualification, and monitoring helps identify critical suppliers and manage risks associated with the supply chain.

4. **Corrective and Preventive Actions (CAPA):** Risk management feeds into the CAPA process within the QMS. When non-conformities,

incidents, or adverse events occur, risk analysis is performed to understand the root causes and determine appropriate corrective and preventive actions to address the risks and prevent their recurrence.

5. **Change Management:** Both risk management and QMS require robust change management processes. When changes are proposed, such as design modifications, manufacturing process changes, or supplier changes, risk assessment is conducted to evaluate the potential impact on product quality, safety, and regulatory compliance.

6. **Post-Market Surveillance:** Risk management and QMS intersect in post-market surveillance activities. Adverse event reporting, complaint handling, and vigilance systems are part of QMS processes that involve risk assessment, analysis, and management to ensure ongoing product safety and regulatory compliance.

7. **Continual Improvement:** Risk management and QMS share a common goal of continual improvement. By analyzing risks and identifying opportunities for improvement, both disciplines drive the enhancement of product quality, safety, and customer satisfaction.

Integrating risk management into the QMS ensures a comprehensive approach to quality and risk throughout the product lifecycle. It helps manufacturers proactively identify and mitigate risks, comply with regulatory requirements, and deliver safe and effective medical devices to patients and healthcare providers.

This table below provides a comparison between risk management and quality management systems, highlighting their key aspects and how they intersect.

TABLE 9.1: COMPARISON BETWEEN RISK MANAGEMENT AND QUALITY MANAGEMENT SYSTEMS

Aspect	Risk Management	Quality Management Systems
Approach	Proactive identification, analysis, and mitigation of risks	Systematic approach to ensure quality and regulatory compliance
Integration	Integrated into all stages of the product lifecycle	Comprehensive management system for quality processes
Design Control	Risk assessment informs design control activities	Design control processes ensure compliance and risk mitigation
Supplier Management	Risk-based supplier selection and qualification	Supplier management processes to ensure quality and reliability
Corrective and Preventive Actions (CAPA)	Risk analysis informs CAPA process	CAPA processes address quality non-conformities and mitigate risks
Change Management	Risk assessment of proposed changes	Change management processes consider risk implications
Post-Market Surveillance	Risk analysis and management in adverse event reporting	Post-market surveillance activities ensure ongoing product safety
Continual Improvement	Identify areas for improvement through risk analysis	Continual improvement efforts to enhance quality processes

9.1 INTEGRATION OF RISK MANAGEMENT WITH QUALITY MANAGEMENT SYSTEMS

The integration of risk management with quality management systems (QMS) is crucial for ensuring the safety, efficacy, and compliance of medical devices. Here are key aspects of integrating risk management with QMS:

1. **Risk-Based Approach:** Risk management and QMS share a common foundation in adopting a risk-based approach. Both disciplines emphasize the identification, assessment, and mitigation of risks to support decision-making and prioritize resources effectively.

2. **Risk Management Procedures:** QMS should include specific procedures and processes for risk management activities. These procedures outline how risk management will be conducted throughout the product lifecycle, including risk assessment, risk analysis, risk control measures, and risk monitoring.

3. **Documentation and Records:** Integrating risk management with QMS requires proper documentation and record-keeping. Risk management activities, including risk assessments, risk analyses, and risk control measures, should be documented and maintained as part of the QMS documentation to ensure traceability and transparency.

4. **Design Control:** Risk management should be an integral part of the design control process within the QMS. Risk assessments and analyses should be conducted during the design and development phases to identify and mitigate potential risks associated with the design, materials, and manufacturing processes.

5. **Risk Control Measures:** The QMS should include mechanisms for implementing and monitoring risk control measures. This involves establishing procedures for implementing risk mitigation strategies, verifying their effectiveness, and updating them necessary to address identified risks.

6. **CAPA Integration:** The QMS should integrate risk management with corrective and preventive actions (CAPA) processes. When non-

conformities, incidents, or adverse events occur, risk analysis should be conducted to understand the root causes and determine appropriate CAPA measures to address risks and prevent recurrence.

7. **Training and Competence:** Integration of risk management with QMS requires training and competence development. Personnel involved in risk management activities should receive appropriate training to understand the principles, processes, and techniques related to risk management.

8. **Continual Improvement:** The integration of risk management with QMS supports the concept of continual improvement. Risk management activities, including the analysis of incidents, near misses, and customer feedback, contribute to identifying areas for improvement within the QMS and driving ongoing enhancements.

By integrating risk management principles and practices into the QMS, organizations can establish a comprehensive approach to quality and risk, ensuring compliance with regulatory requirements, enhancing product safety, and driving continuous improvement throughout the product lifecycle.

9.2 RISK-BASED APPROACHES TO QMS

A risk-based approach to quality management systems (QMS) emphasizes the identification, assessment, and management of risks throughout the product lifecycle. By integrating risk management principles into the QMS, organizations can make informed decisions, allocate resources effectively, and prioritize actions to ensure product safety and regulatory compliance. Here are some key aspects of risk-based approaches to QMS (mentioned in Table 9.2):

1. **Risk Management Planning:** Risk-based approaches to QMS start with a comprehensive risk management plan. This plan outlines the organization's approach to risk management, including the scope, objectives, responsibilities, and methodologies to be used. It sets the foundation for integrating risk management into all QMS processes.

2. **Risk Assessment:** Risk assessment is a critical component of a risk-based QMS. It involves the systematic identification of potential hazards, estimation of risk severity and probability, and evaluation of the overall risk level. Risk assessment helps prioritize actions, allocate resources, and define risk acceptance criteria.

3. **Risk Control Measures:** Based on the results of risk assessments, risk control measures are implemented to mitigate identified risks. These measures can include design modifications, process changes, use of protective measures, training programs, and other preventive actions. Risk control measures are integrated into QMS processes to ensure effective risk management.

4. **Change Management:** Risk-based approaches to QMS emphasize the importance of considering risks associated with changes. Organizations need to assess the potential impact of proposed changes on product quality, safety, and regulatory compliance. Risk assessments guide decision-making during change management processes and help determine the level of validation, verification, and regulatory submissions required.

5. **Performance Monitoring and Improvement:** Risk-based QMS focuses on monitoring product performance and key quality indicators to detect emerging risks. Organizations establish mechanisms to collect and analyze data related to product complaints, adverse events, non-conformities, and other quality metrics. These data inform decision-making and drive continuous improvement initiatives.

6. **Regulatory Compliance:** A risk-based approach aligns with regulatory requirements, as many regulatory bodies emphasize the importance of risk management in ensuring product safety and effectiveness. By integrating risk management into the QMS, organizations can demonstrate compliance with applicable regulations and standards.

7. **Risk Communication:** Effective risk communication is vital in risk-based QMS. It involves clear and transparent communication of risks, both internally within the organization and externally to stakeholders

such as customers, regulators, and healthcare professionals. Risk communication ensures that all relevant parties understand the risks associated with the product and can make informed decisions.

By adopting a risk-based approach to QMS, organizations can proactively identify and mitigate risks, enhance product safety and quality, comply with regulatory requirements, and continuously improve their processes. It enables organizations to allocate resources effectively, prioritize actions, and make data-driven decisions to deliver safe and effective products to the market.

TABLE 9.2: RISK-BASED APPROACHES TO QMS

Aspect	Risk-Based Approaches to QMS
Approach	Emphasizes identification, assessment, and management of risks
Risk Management Planning	Develop a comprehensive risk management plan
Risk Assessment	Systematic identification of potential hazards and risk evaluation
Risk Control Measures	Implement measures to mitigate identified risks
Change Management	Assess impact of changes on product quality and regulatory compliance
Performance Monitoring	Monitor product performance and key quality indicators for risk detection
Regulatory Compliance	Align with regulatory requirements and emphasize risk management
Risk Communication	Transparent communication of risks to stakeholders

9.3 AUDITING AND INSPECTIONS FOR RISK MANAGEMENT

Auditing and inspections play a critical role in assessing the effectiveness of risk management practices within an organization. They help ensure compliance with regulatory requirements, identify areas for improvement, and validate the implementation of risk management processes. Here are key aspects of auditing and inspections for risk management (as mentioned in Table 9.3):

1. **Risk-Based Audits:** Audits should be conducted using a risk-based approach, focusing on critical areas of the organization's risk management processes. The audit scope should include evaluating the effectiveness of risk identification, assessment, control, and monitoring activities.

2. **Compliance Verification:** Audits and inspections verify compliance with applicable regulations, standards, and internal policies related to risk management. They ensure that the organization has implemented and adhered to the required risk management processes and controls.

3. **Documentation Review:** Audits involve reviewing documentation related to risk management, such as risk management plans, risk assessments, risk control measures, and risk management reports. The review assesses the adequacy and completeness of documentation and its alignment with regulatory requirements.

4. **Process Evaluation:** Audits assess the organization's risk management processes, including the effectiveness of risk identification techniques, risk analysis methods, risk evaluation criteria, and risk control strategies. They evaluate whether these processes are consistently followed and meet the organization's objectives.

5. **Verification of Risk Controls:** Audits verify the implementation and effectiveness of risk control measures. This includes evaluating whether identified risks have been adequately addressed, whether controls are

properly implemented and maintained, and whether they are monitored and reviewed regularly.

6. **Performance Monitoring:** Audits assess the organization's monitoring and surveillance activities for risk management. This includes evaluating the adequacy of post-market surveillance, complaint handling, adverse event reporting, and corrective and preventive actions related to risk management.

7. **Non-Conformity Identification:** Audits identify non-conformities and areas of improvement in risk management practices. Non-conformities may include inadequate risk assessments, ineffective risk control measures, gaps in documentation, or non-compliance with regulatory requirements. Corrective actions are then implemented to address these non-conformities.

8. **Inspection Readiness:** Organizations should be prepared for inspections from regulatory authorities. This involves maintaining up-to-date documentation, ensuring compliance with regulations and standards, and having proper record-keeping systems in place to demonstrate effective risk management practices.

9. **Continuous Improvement:** Auditing and inspections provide valuable feedback for continuous improvement in risk management. Findings from audits help identify opportunities for enhancing risk management processes, addressing gaps, and implementing corrective actions to mitigate risks more effectively.

By conducting risk-based audits and inspections, organizations can ensure the robustness of their risk management processes, identify areas for improvement, and demonstrate compliance with regulatory requirements. These activities contribute to the ongoing effectiveness of risk management practices and the overall quality of medical devices.

TABLE 9.3: KEY ASPECTS OF AUDITING AND INSPECTIONS FOR RISK MANAGEMENT:

Aspect	Auditing and Inspections for Risk Management
Approach	Risk-based approach to focus on critical areas of risk management
Compliance Verification	Assess compliance with regulations, standards, and internal policies
Documentation Review	Review risk management documentation for adequacy and completeness
Process Evaluation	Evaluate effectiveness of risk management processes and techniques
Verification of Risk Controls	Verify implementation and effectiveness of risk control measures
Performance Monitoring	Assess monitoring and surveillance activities for risk management
Non-Conformity Identification	Identify non-conformities and areas of improvement in risk management
Inspection Readiness	Maintain readiness for inspections from regulatory authorities
Continuous Improvement	Utilize audit findings for continuous improvement in risk management

9.4 Risk Management and Corrective Actions

Risk management and corrective actions are closely intertwined in the context of quality management systems. Corrective actions are implemented to address identified non-conformities, incidents, or potential risks to prevent their recurrence or mitigate their impact. Here are key aspects of the relationship between risk management and corrective actions:

1. **Risk-Based Corrective Actions:** Corrective actions should be prioritized based on the level of risk associated with the identified non-conformity or incident. Risks are assessed and evaluated to determine the appropriate corrective actions to mitigate or eliminate the risks.

2. **Risk Control Measures:** Corrective actions may involve implementing risk control measures to address identified risks. These measures aim to prevent or reduce the likelihood of the recurrence of the non-conformity or incident by addressing the underlying risks.

3. **Root Cause Analysis:** Risk management techniques, such as root cause analysis, are utilized to identify the underlying causes of non-conformities or incidents. By understanding the root causes, appropriate corrective actions can be implemented to address the identified risks and prevent similar issues in the future.

4. **Risk Assessment of Corrective Actions:** Corrective actions themselves are subject to risk assessment. The potential risks associated with implementing the corrective actions are evaluated to ensure that the actions do not introduce new risks or have unintended consequences.

5. **Effectiveness Evaluation:** Risk management principles are applied to evaluate the effectiveness of corrective actions. The implemented actions are monitored and reviewed to assess whether they have effectively addressed the identified risks and prevented the recurrence of non-conformities or incidents.

6. **Iterative Process:** Risk management and corrective actions are iterative processes. If the implemented corrective actions do not adequately mitigate the risks or prevent the recurrence of non-conformities, further risk assessment and additional corrective actions may be necessary.

7. **Continuous Improvement:** The feedback loop between risk management and corrective actions contributes to continuous improvement. Lessons learned from corrective actions and their effectiveness are integrated into the risk management process to enhance risk assessment, control measures, and overall risk management practices.

By integrating risk management principles into the corrective action process, organizations can ensure that non-conformities, incidents, and associated risks are effectively addressed. This approach supports the ongoing improvement of product quality, regulatory compliance, and patient safety.

9.5 RISK MANAGEMENT AND CONTINUOUS IMPROVEMENT

Risk management and continuous improvement go hand in hand within an organization. Continuous improvement is a fundamental principle of risk management, aiming to enhance processes, mitigate risks, and drive overall organizational growth. Here are key aspects of the relationship between risk management and continuous improvement:

1. **Risk Identification:** Continuous improvement involves actively identifying and assessing risks throughout the organization. This includes engaging stakeholders, conducting regular risk assessments, and promoting a culture of risk awareness.

2. **Risk Evaluation:** Continuous improvement requires a thorough evaluation of risks to determine their significance and potential impact on the organization. Risk evaluation helps prioritize improvement initiatives based on the level of risk exposure and potential benefits.

3. **Risk Mitigation:** Continuous improvement activities often focus on implementing risk mitigation measures to reduce the likelihood or impact of identified risks. These measures can include process enhancements, controls, training programs, or technology upgrades.

4. **Lessons Learned:** Risk management encourages the documentation and analysis of lessons learned from incidents, near-misses, and other risk-related events. These lessons provide valuable insights for continuous improvement efforts, helping to avoid similar risks in the future.

5. **Performance Monitoring:** Continuous improvement relies on effective performance monitoring to track the effectiveness of risk management

controls and mitigation measures. Regular monitoring helps identify areas for improvement and allows for timely adjustments to risk management strategies.

6. **Feedback and Communication:** A culture of continuous improvement fosters open communication channels for sharing risk-related feedback and suggestions for improvement. This can include feedback from employees, customers, regulatory bodies, and other stakeholders involved in the risk management process.

7. **Data Analysis and Metrics:** Continuous improvement is driven by data analysis and metrics related to risk management. By collecting and analyzing data on incidents, non-conformities, and performance indicators, organizations can identify trends, root causes, and opportunities for improvement.

8. **Regulatory Compliance:** Continuous improvement aligns with regulatory requirements and evolving industry standards. Regularly reviewing and updating risk management practices ensures ongoing compliance and helps address emerging risks proactively.

9. **Employee Engagement:** Continuous improvement relies on the engagement and involvement of employees at all levels of the organization. Encouraging employee participation in risk management initiatives and providing opportunities for training and development contribute to a culture of continuous improvement.

By integrating risk management principles into continuous improvement processes, organizations can enhance their ability to identify, assess, and mitigate risks effectively. This approach facilitates ongoing learning, growth, and adaptation to changing environments, ultimately improving overall organizational performance and resilience.

CHAPTER 10

CASE STUDIES AND BEST PRACTICES

10.1 CASE STUDY: RISK MANAGEMENT FOR IMPLANTABLE MEDICAL DEVICES

Background:

A medical device company specializes in manufacturing implantable devices used in orthopedic surgeries, such as joint replacements. They recognized the critical need to implement a comprehensive risk management approach to ensure the safety and effectiveness of their products.

Risk Management Process:

1. **Risk Management Planning:** The company established a dedicated team responsible for overseeing the risk management process. They developed a risk management plan outlining the scope, objectives, and responsibilities for each stage of the process.

2. **Risk Identification:** The team conducted a thorough analysis to identify potential risks associated with their implantable devices. This involved considering factors such as device design, materials, surgical procedures, and potential failure modes.

3. **Risk Analysis:** They systematically analyzed identified risks, assessing their likelihood and severity. They utilized various tools such as fault tree analysis, failure mode and effects analysis (FMEA), and hazard analysis to evaluate the potential impact of each risk.

4. **Risk Evaluation:** The company established risk acceptance criteria based on regulatory requirements, industry standards, and their own

internal guidelines. They compared the assessed risks against these criteria to determine if further risk mitigation measures were necessary.

5. **Risk Control:** To mitigate identified risks, the company implemented appropriate risk control measures. This included refining the device design, improving manufacturing processes, enhancing labeling and instructions for use, and conducting thorough testing and validation.

6. **Risk Assessment and Residual Risk Evaluation:** The team reassessed the risks after implementing the control measures to determine if the risks had been adequately reduced. They documented residual risks and assessed their acceptability based on the established criteria.

7. **Risk Management Review:** Regular reviews of the risk management process were conducted to ensure its effectiveness. The company incorporated feedback from post-market surveillance, clinical data, and feedback from healthcare professionals to improve their risk management strategies continually.

8. **Risk Management Report:** A comprehensive risk management report was compiled, documenting all stages of the risk management process. The report included risk assessments, control measures implemented, residual risks, and ongoing monitoring plans.

Outcome:

By implementing a robust risk management process, the company enhanced the safety and reliability of their implantable medical devices. They effectively identified and mitigated potential risks, ensuring that their products met regulatory requirements and industry standards. The risk management approach enabled the company to provide healthcare professionals and patients with confidence in the safety and performance of their devices.

Lessons Learned:

This case study highlights the importance of a systematic and proactive approach to risk management for implantable medical devices. Key lessons learned include:

- Early integration of risk management in the product development process.

- Utilization of appropriate risk assessment techniques and tools.

- Regular reviews and updates to risk management strategies based on feedback and post-market surveillance.

- Collaboration with healthcare professionals and regulatory bodies to align with best practices and regulatory requirements.

By applying these lessons, other medical device companies can improve their risk management practices for implantable devices and ensure patient safety and product quality.

10.2 BEST PRACTICES IN RISK MANAGEMENT

Here are some best practices in risk management that can be applied across the medical device industry (Figure 10.1):

1. **Risk Management Integration:** Integrate risk management activities into all stages of the product life cycle, from design and development to manufacturing, distribution, and post-market surveillance. This ensures that risk considerations are addressed early on and throughout the product's lifecycle.

2. **Cross-Functional Collaboration:** Establish a cross-functional team comprising professionals from various disciplines, including engineering, quality assurance, regulatory affairs, and clinical experts. This collaboration ensures a comprehensive and holistic approach to risk management.

3. **Risk-Based Decision-Making:** Adopt a risk-based approach to decision-making, where risks are assessed, evaluated, and prioritized based on their severity and likelihood of occurrence. This helps allocate resources effectively and prioritize risk mitigation efforts.

4. **Robust Risk Assessment Techniques:** Utilize appropriate risk assessment techniques, such as FMEA, fault tree analysis, and hazard analysis, to systematically identify, analyze, and evaluate risks. These

techniques provide a structured framework for understanding potential hazards and their potential impact.

5. **Continuous Monitoring and Improvement:** Implement a robust post-market surveillance system to monitor the performance, safety, and effectiveness of the medical devices. Regularly collect and analyze data from adverse event reporting, complaints, and user feedback to identify emerging risks and implement necessary corrective actions.

6. **Regulatory Compliance:** Stay updated with regulatory requirements and standards applicable to medical devices, such as ISO 14971. Ensure that risk management practices align with these requirements to facilitate regulatory compliance.

7. **Documentation and Reporting:** Maintain comprehensive documentation of the risk management process, including risk assessments, risk control measures, residual risks, and ongoing monitoring activities. Regularly review and update risk management reports to reflect any changes or improvements.

8. **Training and Education:** Provide regular training and education to employees involved in risk management to enhance their understanding of risk management principles and techniques. This ensures a consistent understanding of risk management practices across the organization.

9. **Supplier and Contractor Management:** Implement a robust supplier and contractor management process, including assessing their capabilities and performance in risk management. Ensure that suppliers and contractors adhere to the same risk management standards and practices as your organization.

10. **Continuous Improvement Culture:** Foster a culture of continuous improvement, where lessons learned from risk management activities are shared and incorporated into future product development and risk management processes. Encourage employees to identify and report potential risks and provide feedback for ongoing improvement.

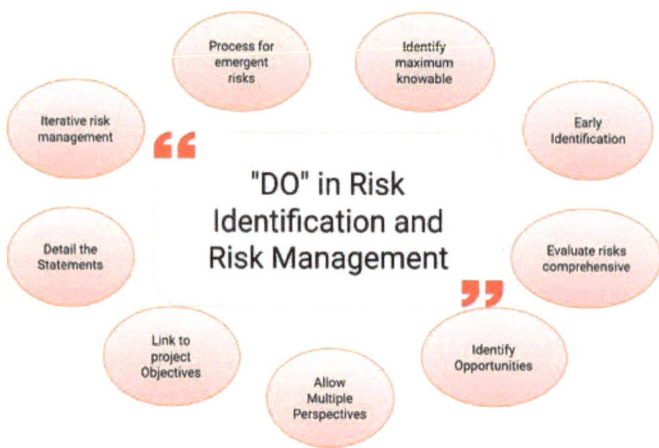

FIGURE 10.1: BEST PRACTICES IN RISK MANAGEMENT

These best practices help ensure effective risk management in the medical device industry, leading to safer and more reliable medical devices that meet regulatory requirements and meet the needs of healthcare professionals and patients.

CHAPTER 11

FUTURE TRENDS AND EMERGING TECHNOLOGIES

Future trends and emerging technologies in risk management in the medical device industry can significantly impact the way risks are identified, assessed, and managed. Here are some key areas of focus:

1. **Artificial Intelligence (AI) and Machine Learning:** AI and machine learning algorithms can enhance risk management processes by analyzing large datasets, identifying patterns, and predicting potential risks. These technologies can assist in early detection of safety issues and enable proactive risk mitigation.

2. **Internet of Things (IoT):** The proliferation of IoT devices in healthcare opens up new possibilities for risk management. Connected medical devices can provide real-time data on their performance, usage, and potential risks, allowing for proactive risk monitoring and management.

3. **Big Data Analytics:** The increasing availability of big data in healthcare enables advanced analytics to identify trends, correlations, and potential risks. By analyzing large volumes of data from various sources, including electronic health records, clinical trials, and adverse event reports, organizations can gain insights into potential risks and take proactive measures.

4. **Digital Health Technologies:** The rapid advancement of digital health technologies, such as wearable devices, telemedicine, and mobile health applications, introduces new risks and challenges. Risk management strategies need to adapt to address data privacy and security concerns, interoperability issues, and the potential impact on patient safety.

5. **Cybersecurity:** With the growing reliance on interconnected devices and digital systems, cybersecurity threats pose a significant risk to the medical device industry. Risk management needs to incorporate robust cybersecurity measures to protect devices and patient data from unauthorized access, hacking, and breaches.

6. **Real-World Evidence (RWE):** RWE, derived from real-world data sources such as electronic health records, claims databases, and patient registries, provides valuable insights into the performance and safety of medical devices in real-world settings. Incorporating RWE into risk management processes allows for more accurate risk assessments and evidence-based decision making.

7. **Human Factors Engineering:** Human factors engineering considers human capabilities, limitations, and interactions with medical devices. Future risk management practices should focus on integrating human factors principles in device design, usability testing, and user training to minimize user-related errors and enhance overall device safety.

8. **Regulatory Changes:** Regulatory bodies continually evolve their requirements for risk management in the medical device industry. Keeping abreast of regulatory changes and aligning risk management processes with updated guidelines is crucial for compliance and ensuring patient safety.

As these future trends and technologies continue to evolve, organizations in the medical device industry should proactively monitor and adapt their risk management practices to address emerging risks and leverage new opportunities for enhancing patient safety and product quality.

11.1 EVOLVING REGULATORY LANDSCAPE AND IMPACT ON RISK MANAGEMENT

The regulatory landscape in the medical device industry is constantly evolving, driven by advancements in technology, changing patient needs, and increasing focus on patient safety. These regulatory changes have a significant impact on risk management practices. Here are some key aspects to consider:

1. **Increasing Regulatory Stringency:** Regulatory bodies worldwide are tightening their requirements for risk management in the medical device industry. This includes more stringent guidelines for risk assessment, documentation, post-market surveillance, and reporting. Organizations must stay updated with these regulatory changes and adapt their risk management processes accordingly.

2. **Harmonization of Standards:** Efforts are being made to harmonize risk management standards globally to streamline regulatory compliance. For example, the International Medical Device Regulators Forum (IMDRF) has developed guidelines to align risk management practices across different jurisdictions. This harmonization facilitates smoother market access and ensures consistent risk management approaches.

3. **Focus on Post-Market Surveillance:** Regulatory authorities are placing increased emphasis on post-market surveillance activities to monitor the safety and performance of medical devices once they are in use. This includes requirements for adverse event reporting, complaint handling, and ongoing risk assessment. Organizations must enhance their post-market surveillance capabilities to meet these regulatory expectations.

4. **Emphasis on Human Factors Engineering:** Regulatory bodies are recognizing the importance of human factors engineering in medical device design and usability. Incorporating human factors considerations into risk management processes is becoming a regulatory requirement in many jurisdictions. Organizations must integrate human factors engineering principles into their risk management practices to address user-related risks effectively.

5. **Integration of Software as a Medical Device (SaMD):** The rise of software-based medical devices, including mobile health applications and AI-powered algorithms, has prompted regulatory bodies to develop specific guidelines for risk management in this domain. Organizations developing SaMD must navigate the unique challenges associated with software-related risks and comply with relevant regulatory requirements.

6. **Global Regulatory Collaboration:** Regulatory bodies are increasingly collaborating and sharing information to harmonize regulatory approaches and align risk management practices. Organizations operating in multiple jurisdictions must navigate complex regulatory landscapes and ensure compliance with the requirements of different regulatory authorities.

7. **Evolving Cybersecurity Requirements:** As medical devices become more connected and vulnerable to cybersecurity threats, regulatory bodies are developing guidelines and regulations to address these risks. Risk management processes must incorporate robust cybersecurity measures to protect devices and patient data from potential cyberattacks.

It is essential for organizations in the medical device industry to monitor regulatory changes closely, engage in proactive dialogue with regulatory authorities, and adapt their risk management practices accordingly. By staying ahead of evolving regulations, organizations can ensure compliance, enhance patient safety, and maintain a competitive edge in the market.

11.2 ARTIFICIAL INTELLIGENCE AND MACHINE LEARNING IN RISK MANAGEMENT

Artificial Intelligence (AI) and Machine Learning (ML) have the potential to revolutionize risk management in the medical device industry. These technologies can enhance the efficiency, accuracy, and effectiveness of risk assessment, monitoring, and mitigation. Here are some key aspects of AI and ML in risk management:

1. **Data Analysis and Pattern Recognition:** AI and ML algorithms can analyze large volumes of data from diverse sources, including clinical trials, electronic health records, adverse event reports, and sensor data. They can identify patterns, correlations, and outliers that may indicate potential risks. This enables proactive risk assessment and early detection of safety issues.

2. **Predictive Analytics:** By leveraging historical data and machine learning algorithms, AI can predict potential risks and their likelihood

of occurrence. This enables organizations to prioritize and allocate resources for risk mitigation strategies, such as design improvements, enhanced testing, or targeted post-market surveillance.

3. **Automated Risk Assessment:** AI can automate certain aspects of risk assessment, reducing human error and improving efficiency. It can assist in categorizing risks based on severity, probability, and impact, enabling more accurate risk prioritization and decision-making.

4. **Real-Time Monitoring and Surveillance:** AI-powered systems can continuously monitor device performance, patient outcomes, and adverse events in real-time. They can identify trends, anomalies, and potential risks, triggering timely interventions or proactive measures to mitigate risks.

5. **Natural Language Processing (NLP):** NLP techniques enable the analysis of unstructured data, such as medical literature, clinical notes, and social media posts, to extract valuable insights related to device safety and risks. NLP algorithms can identify emerging risks, patient concerns, or off-label device usage, facilitating proactive risk management strategies.

6. **Regulatory Compliance Support:** AI can help organizations stay updated with evolving regulatory requirements by analyzing regulatory guidelines, standards, and directives. It can assist in mapping risk management activities to regulatory obligations, ensuring compliance and minimizing regulatory risks.

7. **Decision Support Systems:** AI and ML can provide decision support systems that assist in risk mitigation strategies. These systems can simulate scenarios, evaluate the potential impact of different risk control measures, and optimize risk management strategies based on predefined criteria.

8. **Improved Efficiency and Cost-Effectiveness:** AI and ML technologies can automate repetitive and time-consuming tasks, freeing up resources and allowing risk management professionals to focus on critical

areas. This improves overall efficiency and cost-effectiveness of risk management processes.

However, it is important to note that the use of AI and ML in risk management requires careful validation, robust data governance, and adherence to ethical considerations. Organizations should ensure the transparency, explainability, and reliability of AI algorithms and models to build trust and confidence in their risk management approaches.

Incorporating AI and ML technologies in risk management can significantly enhance the capabilities of organizations in the medical device industry, leading to improved patient safety, enhanced regulatory compliance, and more effective risk mitigation strategies.

11.3 INTERNET OF THINGS (IoT) AND CONNECTED MEDICAL DEVICES

The Internet of Things (IoT) has revolutionized the healthcare industry by enabling the connectivity of medical devices and the exchange of data for improved patient care. However, it also introduces unique risk management challenges that need to be addressed. Here are some key aspects of IoT and connected medical devices in risk management:

1. **Data Security and Privacy:** IoT devices collect and transmit sensitive patient data, including personal health information. Ensuring the security and privacy of this data is crucial to protect patient confidentiality. Risk management strategies should include robust encryption, authentication mechanisms, and secure data storage to prevent unauthorized access and data breaches.

2. **Device Interoperability and Compatibility:** Connected medical devices often need to communicate and exchange data with other devices, systems, or platforms. Ensuring interoperability and compatibility between devices is essential to avoid data discrepancies, misinterpretations, or device malfunctions. Risk management should focus on compatibility testing, standardized communication protocols, and clear documentation of device interactions.

3. **Network Reliability and Resilience:** Connected medical devices rely on network connectivity for data transmission and communication. Ensuring the reliability and resilience of networks is critical to prevent disruptions in device functionality or data loss. Risk management strategies should include network redundancy, backup systems, and proactive monitoring to detect and address network issues.

4. **Cybersecurity Risks:** Connected medical devices are potential targets for cyberattacks, posing risks to patient safety and privacy. Risk management should include robust cybersecurity measures, such as secure authentication, encryption, intrusion detection, and regular security updates. Continuous monitoring and vulnerability assessments are essential to detect and mitigate potential security breaches.

5. **Firmware and Software Updates:** Connected medical devices often require firmware and software updates to address vulnerabilities, improve functionality, or introduce new features. Risk management strategies should include processes for timely and secure updates, ensuring that updates are thoroughly tested and validated before deployment to minimize the risk of device malfunctions or security vulnerabilities.

6. **Regulatory Compliance:** IoT devices in the medical field are subject to various regulatory requirements, including data privacy regulations and medical device regulations. Risk management should incorporate compliance with these regulations to ensure that IoT devices meet the necessary standards for safety, performance, and data protection.

7. **Risk Assessment and Mitigation:** Connected medical devices generate a large volume of data, enabling real-time monitoring and analytics. Risk management should include strategies for continuous risk assessment and mitigation based on the insights derived from IoT data. Proactive identification of potential risks and implementation of appropriate control measures is essential to ensure patient safety and device performance.

8. **User Training and Education:** Connected medical devices may require specific user training and education to ensure proper and safe usage. Risk management strategies should include comprehensive user training programs, clear instructions, and educational materials to empower healthcare professionals and patients with the knowledge to use IoT devices correctly and mitigate potential risks.

The integration of IoT and connected medical devices in healthcare brings numerous benefits but also requires a robust risk management approach to address the unique challenges they pose. By addressing data security, interoperability, cybersecurity, and regulatory compliance, organizations can leverage IoT technologies to improve patient outcomes while effectively managing associated risks (as mentioned in Table 11.1).

TABLE 11.1 : RISKS AND CONSIDERATIONS

Risk Area	Key Considerations
Data Security and Privacy	Encryption, authentication, secure data storage
Device Interoperability	Compatibility testing, standardized protocols
Network Reliability	Redundancy, backup systems, proactive monitoring
Cybersecurity Risks	Secure authentication, encryption, intrusion detection
Firmware and Software Updates	Timely and secure updates, testing and validation
Regulatory Compliance	Data privacy regulations, medical device regulations
Risk Assessment and Mitigation	Continuous assessment, proactive control measures
User Training and Education	Comprehensive training programs, clear instructions

11.4 CYBERSECURITY RISKS AND RISK MANAGEMENT

Cybersecurity risks pose significant challenges in the medical device industry, as the interconnectedness of devices and reliance on digital systems make them potential targets for cyberattacks. Implementing robust risk management strategies is essential to mitigate these risks effectively. Here are key aspects of cybersecurity risks and risk management (as discussed in Table 11.2):

TABLE 11.2 : RISKS AND CONSIDERATIONS IN CYBERSECURITY

Risk Area	Key Considerations
Threat Landscape	Stay informed about evolving cybersecurity threats and trends
Risk Assessment	Conduct comprehensive risk assessments to identify vulnerabilities and potential impact
Security Controls and Measures	Implement technical controls like access controls, encryption, firewalls, and intrusion detection systems
Patch Management	Regularly update and patch software and firmware to address vulnerabilities
Secure Development Practices	Follow secure coding practices and incorporate security throughout the development lifecycle
Incident Response Plan	Develop an incident response plan to effectively respond to and manage cybersecurity incidents.
Employee Awareness and Training	Provide cybersecurity training to employees to enhance their awareness and understanding of risks.

Risk Area	Key Considerations
Supplier and Vendor Management	Assess the cybersecurity practices of suppliers and vendors to ensure their products meet security standards.
Regulatory Compliance	Comply with relevant cybersecurity regulations and standards
Continuous Monitoring and Testing	Continuously monitor and test systems for vulnerabilities and threats
Data Protection and Privacy	Implement measures to protect sensitive data and comply with privacy regulations
Collaboration and Information Sharing	Engage in industry collaborations and information sharing to stay updated on emerging threats and best practices

These considerations should be integrated into a comprehensive risk management framework that includes proactive risk assessment, implementation of security controls, continuous monitoring, incident response planning, and regular evaluation and improvement of cybersecurity measures. By adopting a risk-based approach and incorporating cybersecurity as an integral part of the product life cycle, medical device manufacturers can better protect patient safety and the integrity of their devices and systems.

11.5 Predictive Analytics and Risk Management

Predictive analytics is a powerful tool that can enhance risk management practices by leveraging data and statistical models to make predictions and identify potential risks before they occur. In the context of risk management in the medical device industry, predictive analytics can play a crucial role in proactive risk identification, assessment, and mitigation (as mentioned in Table 11.3).

TABLE 11.3 : KEY CONSIDERATIONS REGARDING PREDICTIVE ANALYTICS AND RISK MANAGEMENT

Risk Area	Key Considerations
Data Collection and Integration	Collect relevant data from various sources, including device data, patient records, adverse event reports, and external data sources.
Data Quality and Cleaning	Ensure data integrity, accuracy, and completeness through data cleaning and validation processes
Statistical Models and Algorithms	Develop and apply statistical models and algorithms to analyze the data and identify patterns and trends
Predictive Risk Identification	Use predictive analytics to identify potential risks and patterns that could lead to adverse events or safety concerns.
Early Warning Systems	Develop early warning systems that can detect signals of potential risks and trigger proactive risk mitigation actions
Proactive Risk Mitigation	Utilize predictive analytics to prioritize and implement risk mitigation strategies based on the identified risks.
Continuous Monitoring	Continuously monitor and update predictive models to adapt to changing risk factors and improve accuracy.
Decision Support	Provide decision support tools that assist stakeholders in making informed risk management decisions based on predictive insights.

Integration with Risk Management Processes	Integrate predictive analytics seamlessly into existing risk management frameworks and processes
Ethical Considerations	Ensure ethical use of predictive analytics, including privacy protection, data anonymization, and compliance with regulations

By harnessing the power of predictive analytics, medical device manufacturers and healthcare providers can proactively identify and address potential risks, enhance patient safety, and optimize risk management efforts. However, it is important to note that predictive analytics should be used in conjunction with other risk management tools and human expertise to ensure a comprehensive and well-informed approach to risk management.

CHAPTER 12

CONCLUSION

I n conclusion, risk management is a critical component of the medical device industry to ensure the safety and effectiveness of medical devices throughout their lifecycle. ISO 14971 provides a comprehensive framework for risk management, guiding organizations in identifying, analyzing, evaluating, and controlling risks associated with medical devices. By following the risk management process outlined in ISO 14971, companies can make informed decisions to mitigate risks and enhance patient safety.

The integration of risk management into various stages of the product lifecycle, including development, manufacturing, distribution, and post-market surveillance, helps identify and address risks at each stage. Additionally, risk management should be closely aligned with quality management systems, as both disciplines share the common goal of ensuring product safety and quality.

Global regulatory requirements and standards further shape risk management practices, necessitating compliance with applicable regulations in different markets. Collaboration and harmonization efforts among regulatory bodies enhance consistency and facilitate international trade of medical devices.

Emerging technologies, such as AI, IoT, and predictive analytics, present new opportunities and challenges in risk management. Leveraging these technologies can improve risk assessment, early detection of potential issues, and proactive risk mitigation.

Case studies and best practices offer valuable insights into real-world applications of risk management, helping organizations understand practical implementation strategies and lessons learned from specific contexts.

Overall, effective risk management is crucial for the medical device industry to ensure patient safety, comply with regulations, and maintain public trust. By adopting a systematic and proactive approach to risk management, organizations can enhance their ability to identify, assess, mitigate, and monitor risks associated with medical devices, thereby contributing to improved patient outcomes and the overall advancement of healthcare.

12.1 KEY TAKEAWAYS

Here are the key takeaways from the discussion on risk management in the medical device industry:

1. Risk management is vital in the medical device industry to ensure the safety and effectiveness of medical devices throughout their lifecycle.

2. ISO 14971 provides a comprehensive framework for risk management, guiding organizations in identifying, analyzing, evaluating, and controlling risks associated with medical devices.

3. Risk management should be integrated into the product lifecycle, including development, manufacturing, distribution, and post-market surveillance.

4. Compliance with global regulatory requirements and standards is essential for risk management in different markets.

5. Emerging technologies, such as AI, IoT, and predictive analytics, offer new opportunities and challenges in risk management, enabling proactive risk identification and mitigation.

6. Case studies and best practices provide valuable insights into real-world applications of risk management, helping organizations learn from practical examples and enhance their risk management practices.

7. Risk management should be closely aligned with quality management systems to ensure the overall safety and quality of medical devices.

8. Post-market surveillance and feedback loops play a critical role in continuous risk management, enabling organizations to monitor and address risks even after devices are on the market.

9. The evolving regulatory landscape and international harmonization efforts impact risk management practices, necessitating compliance with applicable regulations in different regions.

10. Collaboration and information sharing among stakeholders contribute to improved risk management practices and better patient outcomes.

By implementing effective risk management practices, organizations in the medical device industry can enhance patient safety, comply with regulations, and maintain the trust of healthcare providers and patients.

12.2 IMPORTANCE OF PROACTIVE RISK MANAGEMENT

Proactive risk management is of paramount importance in the medical device industry. Here are key reasons highlighting its significance:

1. **Patient Safety:** The primary objective of proactive risk management is to ensure patient safety. By identifying and addressing potential risks early in the product lifecycle, organizations can prevent adverse events, mitigate harm, and protect patients from unnecessary risks.

2. **Regulatory Compliance:** Proactive risk management is essential for regulatory compliance. Regulatory authorities require medical device manufacturers to demonstrate a systematic approach to risk management, as outlined in standards such as ISO 14971. Compliance with these requirements is necessary for market approval and continued market access.

3. **Reputation and Trust:** Proactively managing risks demonstrates an organization's commitment to quality and safety. It helps build and maintain a positive reputation in the industry and among healthcare providers and patients. Trust in the safety and reliability of medical devices is crucial for market success and patient acceptance.

4. **Cost Savings:** Early identification and mitigation of risks can prevent costly recalls, litigation, and damage to an organization's financial health. By investing in proactive risk management, companies can avoid potential financial burdens associated with post-market issues and regulatory non-compliance.

5. **Innovation and Product Development:** Proactive risk management promotes innovation and facilitates the development of safe and effective medical devices. By understanding and managing risks early on, organizations can confidently pursue new technologies and product enhancements, driving advancements in healthcare.

6. **Competitive Advantage:** Organizations that effectively implement proactive risk management differentiate themselves in the market. They gain a competitive edge by demonstrating their commitment to patient safety, quality, and regulatory compliance. This can lead to increased customer trust, market share, and business growth.

7. **Continuous Improvement:** Proactive risk management fosters a culture of continuous improvement within organizations. By regularly evaluating and refining risk management processes, organizations can identify areas for improvement, learn from past experiences, and optimize their risk management practices over time.

Overall, proactive risk management is essential for ensuring patient safety, regulatory compliance, maintaining a positive reputation, and achieving long-term success in the medical device industry. By identifying and mitigating risks early, organizations can protect patients, enhance their competitive position, and drive innovation and growth.

12.3 CONTINUOUS IMPROVEMENT IN RISK MANAGEMENT

Continuous improvement in risk management is a fundamental aspect of maintaining an effective risk management system in the medical device industry. Here are key reasons highlighting the importance of continuous improvement:

1. **Enhancing Patient Safety:** Continuous improvement allows organizations to identify and address new and evolving risks to patient safety. By staying proactive and vigilant, companies can update their risk management strategies and processes to ensure that potential hazards are consistently identified and mitigated.

2. **Adapting to Regulatory Changes:** Regulatory requirements and standards are dynamic and subject to change. Continuous improvement ensures that organizations stay up-to-date with the latest regulatory expectations and incorporate any necessary changes into their risk management practices. This helps maintain compliance and prevent regulatory non-conformities.

3. **Incorporating Lessons Learned:** Continuous improvement enables organizations to learn from past experiences and incorporate lessons learned into their risk management processes. By analyzing incidents, near-misses, customer feedback, and post-market surveillance data, organizations can identify areas for improvement and implement corrective actions to prevent similar issues in the future.

4. **Optimizing Resources:** Continuous improvement helps organizations optimize their resources by identifying inefficiencies, streamlining processes, and eliminating unnecessary steps in the risk management process. This can lead to improved efficiency, reduced costs, and better allocation of resources to critical risk areas.

5. **Fostering a Culture of Quality and Safety:** Emphasizing continuous improvement in risk management fosters a culture of quality and safety within an organization. It encourages employees to engage in risk identification actively, reporting, and mitigation activities, promoting a collective commitment to patient safety and organizational excellence.

6. **Stakeholder Confidence and Trust:** Organizations that demonstrate a commitment to continuous improvement in risk management gain the confidence and trust of stakeholders, including regulatory authorities, healthcare providers, and patients. This can positively impact the organization's reputation, market standing, and long-term success.

7. **Staying Ahead of Emerging Risks:** Continuous improvement allows organizations to anticipate and address emerging risks associated with new technologies, market trends, and changing healthcare practices. By staying proactive and adaptive, organizations can effectively manage these risks and maintain their competitive advantage.

Overall, continuous improvement in risk management ensures that organizations remain responsive, adaptable, and proactive in addressing risks throughout the lifecycle of their medical devices. It helps organizations maintain regulatory compliance, enhance patient safety, optimize resources, and foster a culture of quality and safety. By embracing continuous improvement, organizations can effectively navigate the evolving landscape of risks and maintain their commitment to excellence in risk management.

A. GLOSSARY OF TERMS

Terms	Definitions
Risk	The combination of the probability of occurrence of harm and the severity of that harm
Risk Management	The systematic application of management policies, procedures, and practices to the tasks of analyzing, evaluating, controlling, and monitoring risks.
Hazard	A potential source of harm
Risk Assessment	The overall process of risk identification risk analysis and risk evaluation
Risk Identification	The process of finding recognizing and describing risks
Risk Analysis	The process of comprehending the nature of risks and determining their level of acceptability
Risk Evaluation	The process of comparing the results of risk analysis with risk criteria to determine whether the risk and/or its magnitude is acceptable or tolerable
Risk Control	The process of implementing measures to reduce the risk to an acceptable level
Residual Risk	The risk remaining after risk control measures have been implemented
Risk Acceptance	The decision to accept risk based on a risk evaluation

Terms	Definitions
Risk Management Plan	A document that outlines the approach activities and responsibilities for managing risks throughout the product life cycle
Risk Register	A document that captures and records identified risks including their description severity, likelihood and risk control measures
Risk Mitigation	The implementation of actions or measures to reduce the likelihood or severity of a risk
Post-Market Surveillance	The systematic process of collecting, analyzing and monitoring information on the safety and performance of medical devices after they have been placed on the market
Non-Conformity	A deviation or failure to meet specified requirements or standards
Corrective Action	Actions taken to eliminate the causes of a detected non-conformity or other undesirable situation
Preventive Action	Actions taken to eliminate the causes of potential non-conformities or other undesirable situations
Quality Management System (QMS)	A set of policies, processes, and procedures implemented by an organization to ensure that products or services consistently meet customer and regulatory requirements.
Validation	The process of establishing documented evidence that a system or process, when operated within specified parameters, can perform effectively and consistently.
Verification	The process of evaluating a system or component to determine whether it complies with specified requirements

Terms	Definitions
Risk Benefit Analysis	The process of evaluating and comparing the risks associated with a medical device against its intended benefits to determine if the benefits outweigh the risks
Hazardous Situation	A circumstance in which a medical device has the potential to cause harm
Probability	The likelihood of a specific event or outcome occurring
Severity	The degree of harm that can result from a hazardous situation or event
Risk Management File	A compilation of documents and records related to risk management activities, including risk assessments, risk control measures, and risk management reports.
Risk Management Review	A systematic evaluation of the effectiveness of risk management activities and the identification of any necessary updates or improvements
Risk Communication	The process of sharing information about risks associated with a medical device to stakeholders, such as healthcare professionals, patients, and regulatory authorities.
Risk Residual Limit	The maximum acceptable level of risk after risk control measures have been implemented
Risk Monitoring	The ongoing process of tracking and evaluating the effectiveness of risk control measures and identifying any emerging risks
Adverse Event	Any untoward medical occurrence associated with the use of a medical device, including device malfunctions, injuries, or deaths.

Terms	Definitions
Risk Register Update	The process of periodically reviewing and updating the risk register to reflect changes in the identified risks, their severity, likelihood, and risk control measures.
Risk Management Training	Educational programs and initiatives designed to enhance the knowledge and skills of individuals involved in risk management activities
Risk Management Team	A multidisciplinary group of individuals responsible for conducting risk management activities, including representatives from engineering, quality assurance, regulatory affairs, and clinical disciplines.
Risk Management Documentation	Written records and reports that document the risk management process, including risk assessments, risk management plans, and risk management reports.
Risk Management SOPs	Standard operating procedures that outline the step-by-step processes and instructions for conducting risk management activities in accordance with established policies and regulations

B. RISK MANAGEMENT TEMPLATES AND CHECKLISTS

4. General requirements for risk management		
Item number	**Requirement**	**Complete?**
4.1	**Risk management process**	
	Has the organization ensured the availability of a risk management procedure as part of the design and development of its medical device?	☐
	Does the risk management process extend into the post-production phase (including sterilization, packaging, and labeling where appropriate)?	☐
	Is production and post-production information and data collected and reviewed as part of the risk management process?	☐
	Does the organization's quality management system integrate the risk management process?	☐
4.2	**Management responsibilities**	
	Are top management involved in the overall guidance and effectiveness review of the risk management process?	☐
	Are adequate resources provided for effective risk management activities?	☐

4. General requirements for risk management		
Item number	**Requirement**	**Complete?**
	Are competent individuals trained in the risk management techniques with which they are involved?	☐
	Has top management established a policy for determining acceptable risks and risk levels?	☐
	Does top management participate in periodic review of risk management activities to rectify any weaknesses, implement improvements, and adapt to changes?	☐
4.3	**Qualification of personnel**	
	Are only competent people with the necessary knowledge and experience performing risk management tasks: construction, production, intended use determination, application of medical device?	☐
	Are representatives from various disciplines or functions involved in risk management activity to ensure balanced input?	☐
	Are records to provide objective evidence of competence and training maintained?	☐
	Are personnel records properly maintained with confidentiality and security and without duplication?	☐
4.4	**Risk management plan**	
	Is a properly organized, maintained plan for continual risk management in place?	☐
	Does the plan encourage objective and comprehensive evaluation of risks?	☐
	Is a procedure in place for the development and continued development of the plan?	☐

4. General requirements for risk management		
Item number	**Requirement**	**Complete?**
	Does the plan contain a thorough description of the pertaining device, including a clear thorough statement of intended use?	☐
	Does the plan define a scope to establish the baseline on which risk management activities are built, and involve identification of the medical device and the phases of its lifecycle?	☐
	Does the plan clearly allocate responsibilities and authorities to the respective individuals to ensure accountability?	☐
	Are risk management activities carried out under the plan frequently reviewed by management as an essential responsibility?	☐
	Are the criteria for risk acceptability defined before beginning risk analysis for effective risk management?	☐
	Are the evaluation methods and criteria for acceptability of the overall residual risk decided?	☐
	Is verification activity planned, ensuring that essential resources are available when required?	☐
	Does the plan align with the device's design verification and validation activities?	☐
	Do risk acceptability criteria in the plan derive from your policy of determining acceptable levels of device risk?	☐
	Are the methods for collection and review of production and post- production information to act as input the risk management process properly defined?	☐

\ 4. General requirements for risk management		
Item number	**Requirement**	**Complete?**
	Is a record of changes kept to facilitate audit and review of the risk management process for each particular device?	☐
4.5	**Risk management file**	
	Is the location of all records and other documents applicable to risk management activity properly recorded and maintained, with ready retrieval from a file or file index?	☐
	Is the traceability of records and other documents maintained to help in auditing activities and completion of risk management activities?	☐
	Does the risk management file fully demonstrate that the risk management process is applied to each identified hazard?	☐
	Are identified hazards, or any step-in risk management process such as unspecified or ineffective risk control measures, appropriately controlled?	☐
5.	**Risk analysis**	
5.1	**Risk analysis process**	
	Where applicable, have you checked the available information on risk analysis for a similar medical device on the market?	☐
	Has the organization systematically assessed the previous work for applicability to your current risk analysis?	☐
	Have you ensured that a basic minimum data set is available for traceability, management reviews and audits?	☐

4. General requirements for risk management		
Item number	**Requirement**	**Complete?**
	Have you clarified the scope of your risk analysis and if it verifies completeness?	☐
5.2	**Intended use/reasonably foreseeable misuse**	
	Does the documented intended use include elements like medical condition, patient population, part of the body or type of tissue interacted with, user profile, use environment and operating principle?	☐
	Has the intended user(s) been considered, and whether a lay user or trained professional will use the device?	☐
	Has the use of the medical device in situations that are not foreseen or intended by the manufacturer been considered to a reasonable degree?	☐
	Have future hazards due to potential uses of the medical device, and also reasonably foreseeable misuse, been considered and documented?	☐
5.3	**Identification of characteristics related to safety**	
	Have all characteristics that are qualitative or quantitative and can be related to the operating principle of the device, its intended use, and/or reasonably foreseeable misuse which could affect the safety of the medical device, been documented?	☐

4. General requirements for risk management		
Item number	**Requirement**	**Complete?**
	Have all characteristics been related to the performance of the medical device and to the sterility/measuring function, materials used for parts coming into contact with the patient, usage of radiation for diagnostics or therapeutics, or others?	☐
	Has it been considered whether the limitations of these characteristics, if exceeded, could affect the safety of the device?	☐
5.4	**Identification of hazards/hazardous situations**	
	Have anticipated hazards in both normal and faulty conditions based upon the intended use, reasonably foreseeable misuse, and characteristics related to the safety of the device been identified and documented?	☐
	Have hazardous situations been identified, with associated risks assessed?	☐
	Has the reasonably foreseeable sequence of events that can transform a hazard into a hazardous situation been documented?	☐
	Have typical hazards been listed, demonstrating the relationship with hazardous situations, foreseeable sequences of events, and associated possible harm?	☐
	Is the method of hazard analysis determined, considering whether an expert group, outside sources and product history are used?	☐

4. General requirements for risk management		
Item number	**Requirement**	**Complete?**
5.5	**Risk estimation**	
	Have both components of risk, probability of occurrence and severity of harm, been separately analyzed?	☐
	Is a systematic process in place, including qualitative scales, for categorizing the severity levels and the probability of occurrence of harm, with relevant information recorded within the risk management file and relevant personnel trained in the application of these qualitative scales?	☐
	Are systematic faults, or the sequence of events leading to hazardous situations, continually monitored?	☐
	Are the resulting hazardous situations separately listed, with focus on reducing the risks due to these situations?	☐
	Is quantitative data made available where possible for a new device development or security risk?	☐
	Have risks been evaluated and estimated in a qualitative way – and quantitative, if the data is available?	☐
	Is a mechanism in place for managing risks whose probability cannot be reasonably defined?	☐
6.	**Risk evaluation**	
	Has the acceptability of the risk of the medical device been defined?	☐

4. General requirements for risk management		
Item number	**Requirement**	**Complete?**
	Have estimated risks been evaluated by using the criteria for risk acceptability defined in the risk management plan?	☐
	Have risks been actively investigated to determine which require controls?	☐
	Are risks that need to be controlled identified for further action?	☐
7.	**Risk control**	
7.1	**Risk control option analysis**	
	Has the design and manufacture of the medical device been determined to be inherently safe, with protective measures such as alarms and barriers as appropriate?	☐
	Have risk mechanisms from ISO/IEC Guide 63:2019 been considered and followed?	☐
	Has information for safety, such as written warning or contra- indications and/or training to users or intended users, been provided?	☐
	Are procedures in place to ensure no risk is originating from contamination of components, residues of hazardous substances used in the manufacturing process, or mix-up of parts?	☐
	Are protective measures, such as visual inspection steps in the manufacturing process, applied as appropriate?	☐
	Has a benefit-risk analysis been conducted to determine if the benefit of the medical device to the patient outweighs the residual risk?	☐
	Has the hierarchy of risk control options been explicitly considered?	☐

4. General requirements for risk management		
Item number	**Requirement**	**Complete?**
7.2	**Implementation of risk control measures**	
	Has first verification been conducted to ensure that the risk control measure is implemented in the final design of the medical device or in the manufacturing process?	☐
	Has second verification been conducted to ensure risk control measures as implemented are actually reducing the relevant risks?	☐
	Has the effectiveness of the risk control measures been validated, using a validation study to establish a convincing residual risk evaluation?	☐
	Has the effectiveness of the risk control measures been verified by various testing methods, such as usability testing (IEC 62366-1), testing according to the test standard, clinical investigation of medical devices (ISO 14155), or clinical performance studies for in vitro diagnostic medical devices (ISO 20916)?	☐
	Have verification activities been documented, considering that these activities might happen outside the design stage?	☐
7.3	**Residual risk evaluation**	
	Have the implemented risk control measures made the relevant risk acceptable?	☐
	If the risk is exceeding the acceptability criteria established in the risk management plan, have additional risk control measures been investigated, planned and implemented?	☐

4. General requirements for risk management		
Item number	**Requirement**	**Complete?**
	Are additional risk control measures continually investigated until residual risk does not exceed acceptability criteria?	☐
	Are risks appropriately re-evaluated after implementation of risk controls?	☐
7.4	**Benefit-risk analysis**	
	Has device evaluation proven that the risk does not exceed the criteria for risk acceptability and that the benefit of the device outweighs the risk?	☐
	Does benefit-risk analysis activity exclude economic or business considerations?	☐
	Are properly delineated roles and responsibilities in place for the conducting of benefit-risk analysis?	☐
7.5	**Risks arising from risk control measures**	
	When implementing new risk control measures, alone or in combination, is it actively considered whether they are introducing a new or a different hazard themselves?	☐
	Are steps taken to ensure any risk control measure introduced to reduce one risk is not increasing another risk?	☐
	Has the impact of risk control measures been evaluated?	☐
7.6	**Completeness of risk control**	
	Are all identified hazards and their consequences dealt with?	☐
	Are steps taken to ensure that no hazardous situations are left out of risk analysis activities?	☐

4. General requirements for risk management		
Item number	**Requirement**	**Complete?**
8.	**Evaluation of overall risk**	
	Has the combined impact of all individual residual risks been considered?	☐
	Has the overall residual risk as defined in the risk management plan been evaluated by balancing the overall residual risk against the benefits of the medical device?	☐
	Is all relevant information made available to users about significant residual risks to facilitate the making of informed decisions on their use of the medical device?	☐
	Is all pertinent information on residual risks included in the accompanying documentation, such as IFU/eIFU, product label, user manual, guide?	☐
	Are records of risk evaluation properly kept and maintained, including meeting records and analysis output documents?	☐
	Are senior management involved in consistent risk evaluation and re- evaluation activity?	☐
9.	**Risk management review**	
	Are the final results of the risk management process reviewed after executing the risk management plan?	☐
	Are the results of the risk management review recorded into a risk management report?	☐
	Is the execution of the risk management plan continually reviewed at planned intervals to confirm if the required objective has been achieved?	☐

	4. General requirements for risk management	
Item number	**Requirement**	**Complete?**
	Is the risk management report updated as required during the lifecycle of the medical device according to production and post-production activities?	☐
	Does the risk management report summarize all risk management activities?	☐
	Does the risk management report include traceability of hazards to residual risks? Is this traceability matrix complete and maintained?	☐
	Does the traceability matrix receive review and sign-off by senior management?	☐
	Does the organization determine when subsequent reviews of the execution of the risk management plan need to be performed and when the risk management report needs to be updated?	☐
10.	**Production & post-production activities**	
10.1	**Information collection**	
	Is production and post-production information continually collected and reviewed to evaluate its relevance to safety?	☐
	Are procedures in place for linking information into the risk management review for:	☐
	Manufacturing?	☐
	CAPA?	☐
	Servicing	☐
	Purchasing?	☐

	4. General requirements for risk management		
Item number	**Requirement**	**Complete?**
	Any other pertinent operational areas which demand risk management review?	☐
	Is best industry practice – 'state of the art' – considered, including new or revised standards for the collection and review of this information?	☐
10.2	**Information review**	
	Is production and post-production information related to new hazards or hazardous situations, possible relevance to safety, or the effect on risk estimates and/or the balance between benefit and overall residual risk, continually reviewed?	☐
10.3	**Actions**	
	Is relevant safety information considered and applied as an input for a) continual improvement and modification of the medical device and b) to improve adjoining risk management processes?	☐
	Are the outputs of prior risk management review activity translated into corrective and preventive action?	☐
	What criteria are used to determine if and when risk analysis activity should be revisited?	☐
	Does this activity encompass devices already on the market, as well as those pre-market?	☐

C. RELEVANT STANDARDS AND GUIDELINES

Here are some relevant standards and guidelines related to risk management in the medical device industry:

1. ISO 14971:2019 - Medical devices - Application of risk management to medical devices: This is the international standard that provides a framework for risk management in the design, development, production, and post-market surveillance of medical devices.

2. IEC 62366-1:2015 - Medical devices - Part 1: Application of usability engineering to medical devices: This standard focuses on the application of human factors engineering principles to ensure the usability and safety of medical devices.

3. ISO 13485:2016 - Medical devices - Quality management systems - Requirements for regulatory purposes: This standard outlines the requirements for a quality management system for medical device manufacturers, including the integration of risk management processes.

4. FDA Guidance Documents: The U.S. Food and Drug Administration (FDA) provides various guidance documents related to risk management, including "General Principles of Software Validation" and "Applying Human Factors and Usability Engineering to Medical Devices."

5. IEC 60601-1: Medical electrical equipment - Part 1: General requirements for basic safety and essential performance: This standard

sets forth general requirements for the safety and performance of medical electrical equipment.

6. ISO/TR 24971:2020 - Medical devices - Guidance on the application of ISO 14971: This technical report provides guidance on the application of ISO 14971, including examples and clarification of key concepts.

7. FDA Quality System Regulation (QSR) 21 CFR Part 820: The FDA's QSR outlines the requirements for quality systems for medical device manufacturers in the United States, including the integration of risk management processes.

8. GHTF/SG3/N15:2011 - Risk management throughout the life cycle of medical devices: This guidance document from the Global Harmonization Task Force (now the International Medical Device Regulators Forum) provides guidance on risk management practices throughout the life cycle of medical devices.

9. AAMI TIR45:2012 - Guidance on the use of agile practices in the development of medical device software: This technical information report provides guidance on applying agile development practices to medical device software, including risk management considerations.

10. MDSAP Companion Document: This document provides guidance on implementing a Medical Device Single Audit Program (MDSAP), which aims to harmonize and streamline regulatory audits for medical device manufacturers across multiple countries.

11. ISO 10993: Biological evaluation of medical devices: This standard provides guidance on the biological evaluation of medical devices to assess potential risks associated with materials and interactions with the human body.

12. ISO 11607: Packaging for terminally sterilized medical devices: This standard outlines requirements for packaging systems used for terminally sterilized medical devices, including considerations for risk management in packaging design and validation.

13. ISO 15223-1: Medical devices - Symbols to be used with medical device labels, labeling, and information to be supplied - Part 1: General requirements: This standard provides guidelines for the use of symbols on medical device labels and instructions for use to ensure clear communication of risks and safety-related information.

14. IEC 80001-1:2010 - Application of risk management for IT-networks incorporating medical devices - Part 1: Roles, responsibilities, and activities: This standard addresses the risks associated with the use of information technology networks in healthcare settings and provides guidance on incorporating risk management principles.

15. ISO 31000:2018 - Risk management - Guidelines: Although not specific to the medical device industry, this international standard provides general principles, framework, and guidelines for risk management in any organization, which can be applied to medical device risk management practices.

16. MEDDEV 2.7/1 Rev. 4: Clinical Evaluation: This guidance document provides guidance on the evaluation of clinical data for medical devices, including the assessment of potential risks and benefits associated with the device's clinical use.

17. ASTM F2896: Standard Guide for Integrated Composite Drain Systems for Use on Vented Landfill Gas Collection Components: This standard focuses on risk management considerations for integrated composite drain systems used in landfill gas collection systems.

D. REFERENCES

Here are some references that can be used as sources of information for further reading on risk management in the medical device industry:

1. ISO 14971:2019 - Medical devices - Application of risk management to medical devices

2. IEC 62366-1:2015 - Medical devices - Part 1: Application of usability engineering to medical devices

3. ISO 13485:2016 - Medical devices - Quality management systems - Requirements for regulatory purposes

4. FDA Guidance Documents (available on the U.S. Food and Drug Administration website)

5. IEC 60601-1: Medical electrical equipment - Part 1: General requirements for basic safety and essential performance

6. ISO/TR 24971:2020 - Medical devices - Guidance on the application of ISO 14971

7. FDA Quality System Regulation (QSR) 21 CFR Part 820

8. GHTF/SG3/N15:2011 - Risk management throughout the life cycle of medical devices

9. AAMI TIR45:2012 - Guidance on the use of agile practices in the development of medical device software

10. MDSAP Companion Document

11. ISO 10993: Biological evaluation of medical devices

12. ISO 11607: Packaging for terminally sterilized medical devices

13. ISO 15223-1: Medical devices - Symbols to be used with medical device labels, labeling, and information to be supplied - Part 1: General requirements

14. IEC 80001-1:2010 - Application of risk management for IT-networks incorporating medical devices - Part 1: Roles, responsibilities, and activities

15. ISO 31000:2018 - Risk management - Guidelines

16. MEDDEV 2.7/1 Rev. 4: Clinical Evaluation

17. ASTM F2896: Standard Guide for Integrated Composite Drain Systems for Use on Vented Landfill Gas Collection Components

LIST OF FIGURES

LIST OF TABLES

TABLE 1.1	ANNEXES
TABLE 3.1	RISK MANAGEMENT PROCESS ACCORDING TO ISO 14971
TABLE 4.1	ACCEPTABILITY OF RISK
TABLE 7.1	POST-MARKET SURVEILLANCE PROCESSES
TABLE 7.2	POST-MARKET SURVEILLANCE FEEDBACK LOOP
TABLE 7.3	FEEDBACK LOOP FROM CLINICAL TRIALS AND STUDIES
TABLE 8.1	GLOBAL HARMONIZATION OF RISK MANAGEMENT STANDARDS
TABLE 8.2	REGIONAL HARMONIZATION EFFORTS IN RISK MANAGEMENT
TABLE 9.1	COMPARISON BETWEEN RISK MANAGEMENT AND QUALITY MANAGEMENT SYSTEMS
TABLE 9.2	RISK-BASED APPROACHES TO QMS
TABLE 9.3	KEY ASPECTS OF AUDITING AND INSPECTIONS FOR RISK MANAGEMENT
TABLE 11.1	RISKS AND CONSIDERATIONS
TABLE 11.2	RISKS AND CONSIDERATIONS IN CYBERSECURITY
TABLE 11.3	KEY CONSIDERATIONS REGARDING PREDICTIVE ANALYTICS AND RISK MANAGEMENT